Beefy Calisthenics

Step-by-Step Guide to Build Muscle with Bodyweight Training

Daily Jay

© Copyright 2020 - All rights reserved.

The content contained within this book may not be reproduced, duplicated or transmitted without direct written permission from the author or the publisher.

Under no circumstances will any blame or legal responsibility be held against the publisher, or author, for any damages, reparation, or monetary loss due to the information contained within this book, either directly or indirectly.

Legal Notice:

This book is copyright protected. It is only for personal use. You cannot amend, distribute, sell, use, quote or paraphrase any part, or the content within this book, without the consent of the author or publisher.

Disclaimer Notice:

Please note the information contained within this document is for educational and entertainment purposes only. All effort has been executed to present accurate, up to date, reliable, complete information. No warranties of any kind are declared or implied. Readers acknowledge that the author is not engaged in the rendering of legal, financial, medical or professional advice. The content within this book has been derived from various sources. Please consult a licensed professional before attempting any techniques outlined in this book.

By reading this document, the reader agrees that under no circumstances is the author responsible for any losses, direct or indirect, that are incurred as a result of the use of the information contained within this document, including, but not limited to, errors, omissions, or inaccuracies.

Table of Contents

INTRODUCTION 1

CHAPTER 1: THE SCIENCE OF MUSCLE BUILDING 5

   IS THE GYM REALLY NECESSARY? 6
   THE NATURAL CALISTHENICS BODY 7
   THE IMPORTANCE OF MUSCLES 8
      Hypertrophy: How Muscles Grow 9
      The Role of Hormones in Muscle Growth 11

CHAPTER 2: NUTRITION 13

   CARBOHYDRATES, PROTEIN, AND FATS 14
      Ideal Sources of Protein 17
   CALORIES IN, CALORIES OUT, AND BUILDING MUSCLE 18
      Your Basal Metabolic Rate 19
   IDEAL SOURCES OF NUTRITION: THE MEDITERRANEAN DIET 20
   RISKS OF BAD DIETS 28

CHAPTER 3: REST, RECOVERY, AND CONSISTENCY 31

   THE IMPORTANCE OF REST AND RECOVERY 32
   MAXIMIZE MUSCLE GROWTH WITH REST DAYS 34
   THE ROLE OF PROTEIN IN RECOVERY 38
   THE UNDERESTIMATED IMPORTANCE OF SLEEP 40

CHAPTER 4: PROPER EXERCISE SELECTION 47

   COMPOUND VS. STATIC EXERCISES 47
      Compound Exercises 48
      Static Exercises 49
   WHOLE BODY WORKOUT 50
   PULL EXERCISES FOR UPPER BODY 51
      Pull-Ups 51
      Chin-Ups 52

PUSH EXERCISES FOR UPPER BODY AND CORE 53
    Push-Ups 54
    Dips 55
EXERCISES FOR THE CORE 56
    Leg Raises 57
    Side Planks 58
    Superman 60
LOWER BODY EXERCISES 62
    Squats 62
    Calf Raises 63

CHAPTER 5: NINE FUNDAMENTAL MOVEMENTS TO MASTER 66

PULL-UPS 67
CHIN-UPS 69
PUSH-UPS 70
DIPS 72
LEG RAISES 73
SIDE PLANKS 75
SUPERMAN 77
SQUATS 78
CALF RAISES 80

CHAPTER 6: YOUR 21-DAY WORKOUT PLANS 82

THE IMPORTANCE OF PLANNING 82
    Cardio Exercise and Diet Plan 83
    A Note of Caution 85
POSITIVITY AND MOTIVATION 88
PRE-PLANNING PRINCIPLES 90
BEGINNING WITH THE BASICS 93
21-DAY PLAN: FOUR OR FIVE EXERCISES PER SESSION 96
21-DAY PLAN: NINE EXERCISES PER SESSION 99
CARDIOVASCULAR CONDITIONING 107

CHAPTER 7: PROGRESSION 114

MASTERING THE BASIC LEVELS 115
    Basic Level 1 115
    Basic Level 2 118

> *Basic Level 3* *120*
> TRANSITIONING TO INTERMEDIATE LEVEL 1 122
> > *Intermediate Level 2* *124*
> TRANSITIONING TO ADVANCED LEVEL 1 127
> TRANSITIONING TO ADVANCED LEVEL 2 AND MORE ADVANCED
> CALISTHENICS 129
> > *Pull-Ups and Chin-Ups with Leg Raises* *131*
> > *Horizontal Rows* *133*
> > *Reverse Grip Horizontal Row* *134*
> > *Diamond Push-Up* *135*
> > *Handstand Push-Up* *136*
> > *One-Arm Push-Up/Archer Push-Up* *137*
> > *Straight Bar Dip and Parallel Bars Dip* *139*
> > *Tucked Planche Progressions* *141*
> > *Lateral Lunge* *143*

CHAPTER 8: TROUBLESHOOTING 146

> FIRST, DO NO HARM 146
> YOU ARE UNIQUE 147
> GIVE YOUR MUSCLES TIME TO BUILD 148
> BODYWEIGHT CALISTHENICS Q&AS 149
> THINGS YOU MIGHT BE DOING WRONG 157

CHAPTER 9: MYTHS AND MISCONCEPTIONS 164

CONCLUSION 170

REFERENCE LIST 174

IMAGE SOURCES 186

Introduction

How do you imagine building strong, well-defined muscles? Do dumbbells, barbells, kettle weights, and pushing and pulling weights with cables in a crowded, noisy, unclean gym come to mind? It doesn't have to be that way. Instead, consider the impressive physiques of male Olympic gymnasts: well-shaped bodies from head to toe and sharply defined muscles but not excessive like some muscle-bound weightlifters' builds.

The ideal body is not created by pumping iron; there is an easier, safer, better way without the gadgets, gimmicks, and risks of injury. You are in the right place to learn how to achieve the body of your dreams.

Long before fitness centers came into being, men who wanted to get strong have relied on a regimen of bodyweight exercises—called calisthenics—to build muscle, become powerful, and create a natural-looking overall shape. The key for you to achieve the same results is to become functionally strong with bodyweight calisthenics training.

This book will give you the confidence to get started and keep going with enthusiasm as you see impressive improvements and feel stronger, fitter, and more toned every day.

There's a chapter dedicated to nutrition that will give you guidance on carbs, proteins, and fats and will show how the right diet can help build muscles, while the wrong diet can actually lead to muscle loss. You will become knowledgeable about calories and the various diets that do—and do not—help you manage your weight and build lean muscle mass.

You will also learn how to develop the optimal workout routine to build your ideal body faster and easier than traditional, often painful, weightlifting. You will master the nine fundamental calisthenic movements that use your own bodyweight to strengthen your upper body, core, and lower body to ensure a full-body workout. Our 21-day workout plan will get you started and keep you on track every day for optimal results.

Cardiovascular exercise is an essential component of physical fitness and is credited with helping prevent heart disease, obesity, diabetes, and many other diseases. You will learn to select the right cardio routine and learn how long and how intense your cardio workout should be.

You will learn methods for measuring your progress as you try to maximize the results of practicing bodyweight calisthenic exercises. You will be taught the correct way to perform each exercise and how you can progress quickly, transitioning from beginner to intermediate sooner than you think.

There's a comprehensive troubleshooting section with a Q&A to guide you through issues, problems, and challenges, concluding with a review of the myths and misconceptions that people make when trying to build muscles.

Yet, first, the book will begin with the science of muscle building so that you can understand why proven techniques, good nutrition, and healthy rest and sleep habits form the basis of building muscle and achieving your overall fitness goals.

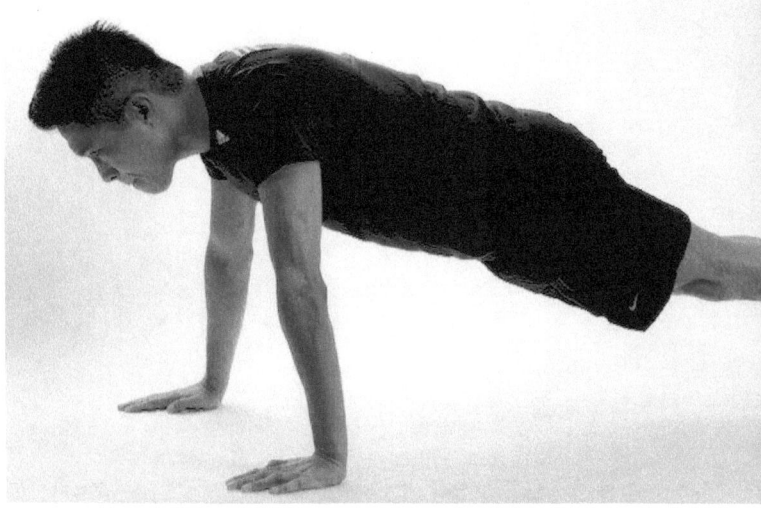

Fig. 1

Chapter 1:

The Science of Muscle Building

There is science behind building stronger, impressive muscles, and by following basic principles, you can start down a path that will lead to tangible, visible results. Knowledge is the key to your success in building a great physique as you grow measurably stronger and look and feel better.

Knowledge begins with understanding what muscle is, what it's made of, how it builds, and how it deteriorates. As you will discover in this chapter, our bodies are designed to build muscle by creating tiny injuries to muscle fibers as you exercise, and these tears, at the cellular level, build new muscle tissue as they heal. But it is important to train correctly so that the correct amount of stress is placed on the muscle fibers.

The right kind and amount of rest and proper recovery time are also critical following each workout so that the muscles can heal and grow. The muscle-building process is also dependent on supplying your muscles, as well as the rest of your body, with the best kind of nutrition.

Is the Gym Really Necessary?

The short answer is, no, gyms aren't necessary, especially not when you can use your own bodyweight to build muscle and get toned with calisthenic exercises. It's more than possible to skip the gym, weights, and machines and still get in great shape.

Further, gyms cost money, and unless you have a fitness center in your home or apartment building, getting to and from the gym takes time. Then, there's the crowding, all those people and too few weights and machines.

Take a good look at many of the guys pumping the big weights in your gym. You can hear them moaning, sighing, and often dropping the weights. That's for your benefit, you know. These are narcissistic people who like to show-off. Is all that noise and drama necessary? Isn't it better to be able to concentrate on your own exercises, not theirs? As you will discover, a good calisthenics workout puts you into the zone of concentration without disturbing distractions.

The Natural Calisthenics Body

Now that you know you don't really need the gym, the next issue is what kind of muscles you want to build. You could purchase a home gym and do weightlifting at home. But why pay for weights when your own bodyweight will provide all the resistance you need for a natural calisthenics body? Look again at the heavy lifters and decide if that kind of bulked-up muscle mass is really what you want.

When our ancestors built muscle through the hard work of their daily lives (chopping, carrying, heaving, fighting, and hunting), they were doing many of the calisthenic bodyweight exercises you'll be learning about here. Their bodies responded naturally and developed the kinds of muscles they needed to live and survive. They became immensely strong, and today, we'd describe their physiques as cut, defined, and powerful.

Respected calisthenics trainer Danny Kavadlo (2017) described how pressing, pulling, and lifting in their daily lives was a hardwired part of their DNA and that the naturally-achieved "calisthenic body is a uniquely impressive physique," which is rippled and muscular with good balance, erect posture, and no superfluous body fat. Contrast this with the weightlifters who are stooped, curved, over-bulked, and muscle-bound. Sure, they're strong, but they've become dysfunctional, unlike the naturally built body that has strength, flexibility, resilience, and good tone.

The Importance of Muscles

We're all aware of our muscles, whether it's when we step out of the shower and see ourselves in the mirror or when we feel the warm glow in our arms, shoulders, chest, abs, and legs after resistance exercises. We're also aware of our muscles when we've overdone exercise or any form of lifting, and our overworked muscles are screaming out with pain. However, muscles are not just for lifting, walking, running, and jumping: our muscles affect our overall health, our metabolic rates, and even our longevity. Having good lean muscle mass is a key component of your well-being, apart from your goals of building muscles and increasing strength.

While there are various types of muscles in our bodies, including the myocardium (heart muscle) and the diaphragm that supports breathing, we're focusing on the 650 skeletal muscles. These are the muscles we see and feel and that contract each time they receive a signal from motor neurons, which are the nerves that connect the muscles to the spinal cord and brain. The better the communication between motor neurons and muscles, the greater the strength of the muscles.

Hypertrophy: How Muscles Grow

Every skeletal muscle is made up of thousands, or millions, of tiny muscle fibers; each fiber is actually a muscle cell built of links known as sarcomeres, which are the foundation of muscle fibers that contract to actually make you move. Each muscle is constructed of these sarcomeres, which contain thread-shaped contractive components called myofibrils, myosin, and actin. When your brain sends a signal for a muscle to contract, it activates the contractile fibers, notably actin and myosin, within the sarcomeres.

The growth of skeletal muscles is called hypertrophy. It's a complex process that begins with the myosin and actin fibers building up the sarcomeres, which, in turn, build up muscle fibers, and ultimately, grow the muscle itself.

According to physiology professor Len Kravitz, PhD, and grad student Young Kwon at the University of New Mexico's Exercise Science Program (2004), when muscle tissue is subjected to intense exercise, there is trauma inflicted on the muscle fibers, defined scientifically as injury or damage to muscle organelles. As a result, satellite cells on the outside of the muscle fibers reconstruct the damaged tissue by fusing with the muscle cells. This action builds the muscle cells, enlarging the muscle fibers; this is the muscle growth process of hypertrophy.

This repair process begins after intense workouts, and with each repair, the muscle fibers become slightly thicker so that, over time, the muscles become visibly larger as well as stronger. Muscle gain occurs if the muscle protein fusion is greater than muscle protein loss or breakdown. Muscle growth is enhanced by additional cell nuclei being added to the muscle fiber cells. Importantly, the repair and growth process of muscle cells and fibers only takes place *during rest after* working out; growth never occurs *during exercise*.

There are three elements that contribute to muscle growth, which include:

1. **Muscle Tension**, which is created by stress that is more intensive than muscles are accustomed to.
2. **Muscle Damage**, which results from the stress of extreme muscle tension.
3. **Metabolic Stress**, which is a process where muscle cells become swollen by the addition of the energy-supplying glycogen, creating the pumped-up sensation. (To be clear, this muscular swelling or pumping-up is temporary, as the actual muscle growth occurs after the exercise when the muscles are in their rest-and-recover phase.)

The Role of Hormones in Muscle Growth

Hormones play an important role in muscle regeneration and growth. You have probably heard about the male hormone testosterone, which is pivotal, as is another hormone called insulin growth factor. Most of the body's testosterone is dedicated to various bodily functions, but during resistance strength training, some testosterone is released and is able to activate muscle cell receptors. The role of testosterone, in this situation, is to increase muscle protein growth, slow the breakdown of protein, and direct neurotransmitter chemicals to damaged muscle cells to activate growth of new muscle tissues.

Insulin growth factor hormone further encourages muscle growth and glycogen release for energy and sends amino acids, which are the building blocks of protein, to the skeletal muscles.

Do these findings suggest that you should ingest hormone supplements to increase the effects of calisthenics? Most likely, not. Medical professionals generally advise not taking hormones without close medical supervision and only when blood tests confirm a deficiency. Your increase in muscle size and strength should come from natural workouts and not from taking potentially risky hormone supplements.

Okay, the scientific part is over and behind us. Now that you are armed with the knowledge of how your muscles grow, you are better able to appreciate the vital role nutrition plays in rebuilding and strengthening muscle fibers and cells. It's time to get you on the right track to eat more nourishing, healthier meals without having to give up your enjoyment of eating so that you can bulk up muscle mass while losing body fat. Ready? Let's start eating right.

Chapter 2:

Nutrition

Nutrition is the process of eating, and the *quality* of nutrition is a function of what we eat, how well we digest and assimilate it, and how it affects us. The expression, "You are what you eat," pretty well sums up the concept of nutrition. Of course, it's not that simple. Our gastrointestinal system digests and breaks down foods into basic components so that assimilation does not take place at the granola or Twinkie level but at a more fundamental chemical level. Still, each food we eat has its own nutritional values, calories, and other components that our bodies process and react to. Some foods we eat may also contain chemicals or ingredients that can be potentially harmful.

Good nutrition is everyone's business, since our health, well-being, and longevity depends on it, but it plays a specifically pivotal role for those wanting to build lean muscle mass and get into good physical shape. As you learned in the previous chapter, muscles grow by repairing the cellular damage resulting from calisthenics and other resistance activities, and this growth requires an adequate supply of the amino acids, proteins, and other essential nutrients the repairers utilize. Learning the essentials of nutrition and constructing an ideal diet for optimal overall health and disease prevention is vital in your quest to build a strong, well-defined muscular body.

Carbohydrates, Protein, and Fats

The energy values of the foods we eat are expressed as calories; a calorie is the amount of energy needed to heat one gram of water by one degree Celsius. Every gram of carbohydrates contains four calories, and every gram of protein also contains four calories. Fats (including oils) are different; nature designed fats for storage, so each gram of fat contains nine calories. Carbohydrates and fats have the primary roles of providing energy, while protein rebuilds cells. Indeed, proteins rebuild every one of the trillions of cells in our bodies from muscles to red corpuscles in our blood.

Now, let's look at the three fundamental food groups. We'll begin with a normal basic diet. The daily number of calories needed to gain, maintain, or lose weight is based on current bodyweight, so take an average adult male who needs 2,000 calories per day to maintain a current, normal weight (that is, not overweight or obese). Our source for the following diet is Kathy Lee Wilson (2018), a certified trainer and athlete, and she recommends that:

Quality carbohydrates should account for between 45% to 65% of total caloric intake. To build lean muscle, you will be at the lower end of the scale so that you can leave room for more protein. Most people are surprised that carbohydrates are so important, but we're basing this need on quality carbohydrates, including the vegetables, fruits, berries, whole grains, and cereals that are in the Mediterranean diet, which you'll read about below.

Lean proteins can range from as low as 10% up to 30% of total daily calories. In seeking lean muscle mass, you will be closer to the 30% protein level. The protein that everyone needs to repair cells throughout the body, including restoring blood cells, body organs, skin, hair, and nails, is only part of the equation. Your body will need additional protein to repair and build the skeletal muscle fibers and cells that are broken down during your bodyweight calisthenic exercises. Sources of protein are lean chicken, turkey, fish, low-fat milk and yogurt, and good plant-based proteins, such as nuts, beans, seeds, grains, and cereals.

Healthy fats may account for 25% to 35% of your daily caloric intake, and with the great need for protein to build muscle, your fats may be on the lower end, closer to 25%. The good news is that you will be getting the healthy fats you need for good health from other parts of your diet, including fish, olive oil, nuts (like walnuts and almonds), avocados, and flax seeds. Because fats contain more than twice the calories of proteins and carbohydrates (nine calories per gram vs. four per gram), it doesn't take much to reach that 25% goal for healthy fats.

So, given the above considerations, to optimize building lean muscle, your caloric ratio target should be close to:

- ➤ 45% quality carbohydrates
- ➤ 30% lean protein
- ➤ 25% healthy fats

How many calories does this equal? That depends on your daily caloric input. As we stated above, an average adult male needs 2,000 calories to maintain weight. Remember, there are four calories in each gram of carbohydrates and protein, and nine calories in each gram of fat. On the basis of 2,000 calories per day, that means:

- ➤ **Quality carbohydrates** are 45% of daily intake = 900 calories per day (425 grams)
- ➤ **Lean proteins** are 30% of daily intake = 600 calories per day (150 grams)
- ➤ **Healthy fats** are 25% of daily intake = 500 calories per day (56 grams)

(Look for the *Fitness Calculator* at the beginning of this book, which you can download and use to determine your daily protein and calorie requirements to build strong, lean muscles.)

Ideal Sources of Protein

These foods are good sources of protein:

Food	Serving Size	Calories	Protein (grams)	% Daily 150 gms
Eggs (large)	1 (50 gm)	70	6	4%
Barley, Peas, Lentils, Rice	2 oz (dry)	180	7	5%
Beans, Chickpeas	4 oz	120	7	5%
Nuts (peanuts, walnuts, cashews)	1 oz	170	8	6%
Skim Milk	8 Oz	80	10	8%
Greek Yogurt (0% fat)	6 oz	100	19	14%
Sardines	3 oz	200	22	15%
Chicken, Turkey, Beef (lean)	4 oz	106	24	16%
Tuna (one can)	4 oz	260	26	17%

Calories In, Calories Out, and Building Muscle

As mentioned, a calorie is the amount of energy needed to heat one gram of water by one degree Celsius. What science has proved unequivocally is that weight is gained, lost, or maintained based on *calories in* (ingested) and *calories out* (burned). While no two people digest, metabolize, and assimilate foods at an identical rate, the physics tells us that if your caloric *intake* exceeds your caloric *output*, you will retain the difference, either as muscle (if you work hard at building muscles, that is) or, as is more typically the case, as fat.

If you follow this book's guidance and perform the bodyweight calisthenic exercises, you will not gain weight or fat when you increase your protein intake or even consume more calories than normal. But protein alone won't do the work of muscle building for you. Those four calories per gram will be stored as fat if they aren't assigned to rebuilding muscle fibers and cells that have been stressed and damaged by your good resistance workouts. A diet composed of a 30% daily intake of protein is ambitious and will require increasing normal servings of high-protein foods. These calorie counts you are seeing are approximate, and since no two people have an identical metabolic rate, only through trial and error can you ensure you are managing your weight effectively.

Your Basal Metabolic Rate

When you are at rest without movement or stress, your metabolism is at its lowest level; this is called your basal metabolic rate (BMR). It refers to the minimal number of calories your body needs to survive and sustain itself under the least challenging conditions. Imagine your metabolic rate while you've been lying down for hours, doing nothing. As you are aware, your body is still using calories while you are at rest to perform involuntary functions to support your heartbeat, breathing, digestive organs, brain function, and central nervous system, and, of course, to repair damaged muscle fibers.

While you cannot raise or influence your BMR through activity, it can be raised when lean muscle mass is increased. As a consequence, you can actually burn more calories when at rest, even when you are asleep. Muscle mass has an appetite for calories that supply energy to the continuing rebuilding process, which happens when muscles are resting.

According to Bodybuilding.com ("Calculate Your Basal Metabolic Rate," 2020) the total calories you use every day is known as the "total daily energy expenditure," and it factors in your BMR plus all the activities you perform over the course of a 24-hour day. The total expenditure depends on your activity level, age, and gender. Activity includes everything you do physically and mentally (you may be surprised to learn that your brain accounts for about 3% of your bodyweight but uses around 15% of your caloric energy).

Ideal Sources of Nutrition: The Mediterranean Diet

Nutritionists may have different dietary preferences, but they tend to agree on this basic principle: The best, healthiest diet is based on groups of real foods. What are real foods? They're unprocessed, close to their natural form, rich in nutrients, and free of preservatives, sugar, and other highly refined carbohydrates. Another major agreement is that diets should limit foods containing saturated and trans fats.

Among many ways to eat naturally, the **Mediterranean diet** has emerged in recent years as the ideal diet for keeping healthy, maintaining weight, and generally feeling better. And while this diet is not specifically targeted to building lean muscle, you are free to shift the emphasis to muscle-building protein while keeping within the Mediterranean diet guidelines.

This diet is based on the eating practices of those who live in southern France, Italy, Greece, and other regions close to the Mediterranean basin. It has been shown that the residents of these regions live longer and are healthier compared to those in the rest of the world. They tend to avoid obesity and sedentary lifestyles, being active throughout their lives.

They eat a healthy, balanced, natural diet in moderate portions. You will appreciate the pleasures these practitioners experience from eating real, delicious, minimally processed, and wholesome foods. There's no need to become a vegetarian or vegan; with the Mediterranean diet, you can benefit from a combination of plant-based and animal-based foods.

- ➤ **Plant-based foods** provide essential vitamins, minerals, nutrients, moderate amounts of healthy unrefined carbohydrates, some protein, and healthy fats. Plant-based foods include a wide range of vegetables, fruits, nuts, seeds, beans, whole grains, cereals, and vegetable oils.
- ➤ **Animal-based foods** are essential sources of protein and are higher than vegetables in the muscle-building proteins you need. Yet, they should be consumed in moderation and only when lean. Animal-based foods can include fish, low-fat dairy products, and eggs, which are all high-quality proteins that offer a good source of nutrients.

Let's take a closer look at the groups of **plant-sourced** foods within the Mediterranean diet.

1. **Vegetables** are low in calories and carbohydrates, yet are a storehouse of vitamins, minerals, nutrients, beneficial fiber, and even a moderate supply of protein.

Vegetables the Mediterranean diet encourages you to eat include broccoli, bell peppers, and asparagus, which are low in carbohydrates and calories and supply vitamins K and C as well as fiber and antioxidants. These same nutrients are provided by carrots, Brussels sprouts, cucumbers, beets, and kale. Tomatoes, technically a fruit, contain vitamin C and other nutrients.

In fact, almost all vegetables you'll find at the grocery store are low carbohydrate sources of vitamins, minerals, and antioxidants. Also look for artichokes, celery, cabbage, leeks and onions, Swiss chard, green zucchini, and yellow squash. Experts say that a mix of colors is ideal for supplying different minerals.

2. **Fruits and berries** are nutritious as well as naturally sweet and delicious.

Apples are filling and high in fiber, antioxidants, and vitamin C. They're an ideal healthy dessert or a nutritious snack between meals. Bananas are a great source of the electrolyte potassium, vitamin B6, and fiber. Blueberries have these same nutrients and are also a good source of antioxidants.

Avocados are also in the fruit category but are low in carbohydrates and high in nutritious polyunsaturated avocado oil, potassium, and vitamin C. Other good sources of vitamin C and fiber are oranges, strawberries, grapes, and most other fruits, melons, and berries.

3. **Grains and cereals** have been with us since early hunter-gatherers harvested wild wheat and later when the first farmers began to cultivate wheat, rye, barley, rice, and other grains. In a nutritious diet, grains are whole, rather than refined, retaining the bran, fiber, minerals, and vitamins.

    Brown rice, whole-grain breads and cereals (unsweetened), and quinoa are the most popular healthier grains and contain good levels of magnesium, vitamin B, and fiber. Be aware that "multi-grain" does not mean whole grain; read the labels and stick with unpolished, unrefined grains, cereals, and whole-grain breads.

    Oatmeal is credited with lowering LDL (bad) cholesterol, thanks to its beta-glucans and soluble fiber content. Opt for regular, not pre-cooked oatmeal, since it's higher in nutrients and only takes three minutes to cook.

    Grains and cereals provide moderate levels of protein, but given their high carbohydrate levels, those on medically-recommended low carbohydrate diets may need to limit their grain consumption.

4. **Beans and legumes** are within a family of plant foods called pulses. We're most familiar

with the dried variety, but peas and string beans are pulses, too. For their small size, beans are very high in protein and other key nutrients.

Beans include pinto beans, kidney beans, chickpeas, black beans, lima beans, navy beans, cannellini beans, and soybeans. There are also split peas and lentils. All provide about 7 to 8 grams of protein in a ¼ cup serving (measured dry). You may use the pre-cooked canned versions or begin with dry. (If using dried beans, be sure to presoak before cooking.)

In addition to protein, beans provide complex carbohydrates, fiber, folate, iron, phosphorus, and linoleic and oleic unsaturated acids. Clinical studies cited by Harvard's T.H. Chan School of Public Health (2020) show the phytochemicals in beans help reduce the risks of cardiovascular disease, digestive diseases, diabetes, obesity, and cancer.

5. **Nuts and seeds** are used mostly in snacks, as additives to cereals, and when baking bread, and they are a surprisingly good source of nutrients.

Nuts, including almonds, walnuts, peanuts (actually a legume), pecans, and cashews, are high in beneficial antioxidant oils and fiber. Nuts are an above-average source of protein, copper, magnesium, folate, potassium, vitamins

B6 and E, and niacin. Nuts have been shown to help prevent heart disease, diabetes, and cancer.

Seeds include familiar pumpkin seeds, sunflower seeds, chia, and flax seeds, which have become popular recently and may be sprinkled on cereals and fruits to add fiber, magnesium, calcium, and antioxidants.

6. **Olive oil** and most other plant-derived oils are an ideal, beneficial source of necessary fats.

    The molecular structure of olive oil is primarily monounsaturated oleic acid, an unsaturated fat that studies cited by Joe Leech (2018) in Healthline.com show is good for heart health, especially preventing the build-up of LDL (bad) cholesterol, which can clog arteries. Findings also credit olive oil with good levels of antioxidants and anti-inflammatories. It can reduce your risk of developing diabetes, strokes, and Alzheimer's disease.

    Be sure to use extra virgin olive oil, which is the least processed and most nutritious form. Many other plant-based oils, including soybean, sunflower, corn, and safflower, are polyunsaturated and are also beneficial. Be careful of a few plant-based oils that are high in saturated fats, such as coconut oil.

Now, let's look at **animal-sourced** foods that are part of the Mediterranean Diet.

1. **Meats**, in limited quantities, are an excellent source of muscle-building protein.

   The meats you choose should be on the lean side, including white meat chicken, white meat turkey, lean pork, and lean beef, which is a good source of iron. Be careful to avoid meats marbled with saturated fats, which are to be avoided for cardiovascular health as well as to manage caloric intake.

   Portions of meats should be smaller than you may think. Nutritionists and the American Heart Association (2020) propose the serving of lean meat should be about the size of a deck of cards or three to four ounces. But with a goal of building bigger, stronger, and leaner muscle mass, you may need to increase the portion size of lean meat but not too much. There are plenty of healthy proteins in plant-based foods and in fish.

2. **Fish** is a highly recommended source of quality protein and of valuable nutrients.

   Ideally, your diet will include at least two servings of fish per week. Salmon, cod, sole, seabass, tuna, sardines, swordfish, and mackerel are excellent protein sources. The fats and oils in these cold-water fish are unsaturated. Fish also contain valuable omega-3 fatty acids and iodine.

There have been studies that link diets rich in seafood with living longer and healthier with less chance of developing heart disease, depression, and anxiety.

3. **Dairy** products, including milk, cheese, and yogurt supply good amounts of protein plus vitamins.

   You should limit your selection to fat-free or low-fat milk and yogurt and limit your overall consumption of cheese. Try to avoid or limit full-fat cheeses and cream, which are high in saturated fats.

   Greek and Icelandic yogurts are increasing in popularity due to higher protein levels compared to traditional yogurts, thanks to the straining process that removes excess water.

4. **Red wine** is generally included in the Mediterranean diet, and studies point to healthier hearts and health when the consumption is moderate.

   Some findings suggest that moderate drinkers of red wine and other forms of alcohol are better off than non-drinkers and heavy drinkers. But caution is advised. Moderate for adult men means no more than two 5-ounce glasses of wine, two servings of 1.5 ounces of alcohol, or two 12-ounce servings of beer per day. Doctors advise that if you do not currently drink alcoholic beverages, you should not start.

You may be wondering about eggs. Despite warnings issued decades ago about the cholesterol levels in eggs, nutritionists now rate eggs high on the nutritional chart and recommend up to two eggs per day as a rich source of protein and nutrients.

Now that we've covered the ideal diet for overall health and for building lean muscle mass, we can conclude this chapter with a brief look at the negatives of bad diets.

Risks of Bad Diets

We humans evolved over the millennia, eating a variety of the foods you have just read about in the Mediterranean diet: all-natural, unprocessed or minimally processed, diverse, providing the full range of essential amino acids, full of proteins, and containing healthy carbohydrates and oils. They did not eat greasy, fried foods, overly processed foods containing artificial preservatives, foods with added sugar or other refined carbohydrates, or food full of saturated and hydrogenated fats and trans fats.

They did not eat junk food, and neither should we.

Take the hamburger as an example of how foods can be good and bad, depending on the ingredients.

Imagine a hamburger with two simple ingredients: 95% lean unprocessed chopped meat and a whole-grain bun. The lean meat is supplying about 22 to 24 grams of protein, or 16% of your daily need, plus a small amount of fat. The whole-grain bun adds fiber, vitamins, and minerals that come from the bran layer, plus needed healthy carbohydrates and (surprise!) 2 or 3 grams of protein.

In contrast, take the typical hamburger from a fast-food joint: fatty meat loaded with calories and unhealthy saturated fats, and with fewer grams of protein, since the amount of protein-rich lean meat is less. The bun contributes to the empty calories, too, with over-processed white bread, which is made from refined white flour that has had its natural nutrients removed. Like most white breads, its ingredient list is filled with flavor enhancers, stabilizers, and preservatives.

You can see the huge difference between these two hamburgers, and how one (the healthy version) gives your body what it needs to produce lean muscle.

Beyond that, an unhealthy diet is full of sugar, which is a source of excessive empty calories and is present in many foods and beverages, such as soft drinks and sports beverages. Read the labels and learn to give up sugar-laden foods and drinks.

Fried foods are bad news. The breaded coating absorbs cooking oils, which can become toxic through reheating with trans fats. Like our hamburger example, frying good lean foods deprive them of all their benefits.

Frying potatoes, chicken, and fish add hundreds of fat calories. A donut exemplifies a bad diet of unnecessary, overused oils and trans fats, plus loads of sugar.

Become aware of which foods are more natural and which are overly processed. Get in the habit of reading labels and asking yourself, "Do I want to eat all that sugar and those chemicals?"

You have a good start on developing the right diet, and it's time now to move on and learn much more about the value of rest, recovery, and consistency.

Chapter 3:

Rest, Recovery, and Consistency

Doing calisthenic exercises and nothing else won't allow you to build the lean body you want. Rest and recovery (along with diet) are just as important. The optimization of recovery and rebuilding, through the discipline of consistency, within your daily, weekly, and long-term routines is key to your success in fine-tuning your muscle mass and body.

As you prepare to begin a serious bodyweight calisthenics program and are committed to achieving your bodybuilding goals, the first step (perhaps the biggest step) is mental: Your commitment to perform the exercises, as instructed, on a regular, consistent basis and, just as importantly, to observe the discipline of rest and recovery.

If you just completed a marathon, would you consider hitting the road again tomorrow and running another 26.2 miles? Of course, you wouldn't. Beyond the sheer fatigue, there would be something important—essential—going on in your body. Thousands of muscle fibers are beginning to repair the damage you just imposed on your muscles, and you are recovering from the stress many of your body's organs and functions experienced. Even if you woke up feeling great, your body isn't prepared or ready for more exercise. The same principles apply to serious resistance exercise.

Further, protein also plays a role in helping to build muscles bigger and faster through recovery. And rest and recovery mean nothing if you're not getting a good night's sleep every night.

The Importance of Rest and Recovery

Recovery shouldn't be an afterthought, something you underestimate, or a part of your calisthenics plan you ignore. That's why we want you to understand the great importance of rest and recovery *before* you even get into the actual body weight calisthenics techniques. It's natural to believe that the calisthenics movements you'll be performing are all that matter. But the truth is that all the hard work you do on workout days can be wasted if it's not followed by adequate rest and recovery time. Some athletes actually feel a sense of guilt on days when they don't exercise hard or at all but this is contrary to the fact that adequate recovery time is needed if your damaged cells, fibers, and muscles are to repair and grow in size and strength.

Workouts break down muscle fiber and cells, cause loss of fluids, and deplete stored muscle glycogen energy. During recovery, the body is able to repair and rebuild the muscles and other damaged tissues, replace missing fluids, and recharge the energy supply. But without rest, recovery can't take place, and the body will continue to break down. Closely scheduled hard workouts coupled with no rest and recovery can become detrimental to health and well-being.

Overtraining syndrome is a potentially serious downside to not providing yourself adequate recovery time. In the online fitness journal, *Very Well Fit*, exercise physiologist and sports medicine consultant Elizabeth Quinn (2020) explains that overtraining syndrome occurs from training beyond the body's ability to recover. The result is a reduction in strength and conditioning, rather than growth. Symptoms of overtraining syndrome can include compulsive exercise, reduced immunity (leaving the person susceptible to infections, colds, and flu), continuing sore muscles, aching joints, and a reduction in exercise performance, such as fewer push-ups and pull-ups than normal. Other symptoms may include a loss of energy, irritability, insomnia, and a loss of enthusiasm for workouts.

You can self-diagnose for overtraining by checking your resting heart rate each morning, just after waking. Under normal conditions, your heart rate should be fairly consistent from day to day, but if you record a distinct increase in the resting heart rate, it may indicate that full recovery from the previous workout has not been achieved, and it will be important to make that day one of rest and recovery. Depending on the degree of overwork, several rest days may be necessary. Don't rush it; stay well-hydrated and do not exert yourself. In extreme cases, when overtraining has occurred over a sustained period, it may take several weeks of taking it easy and reducing stress.

Now, let's look at how much rest and recovery is needed.

Maximize Muscle Growth With Rest Days

Recovery takes place in stages, each of which plays a role in resting and rebuilding your muscles. In the hours after completing an intense resistance session, the recovery process enters its first phase, referred to as short-term or active recovery, where you can be performing low-intensity walking or light lifting activities (including housework, gardening, or hiking at a comfortable speed). These light activities should continue into the next day, keeping you active but without exerting yourself. You will also be recharging protein, fluids, and energy stores.

During this active recovery phase, many things are happening inside of you. The strained and damaged muscle cells that you challenged during your workout are going through the recovery process and muscles, ligaments, and tendons are being repaired. Chemicals, including lactic acid, that have built up in the muscle cells are removed. You should allow a minimum of one rest day after a moderate calisthenics workout and at least two consecutive rest days after a hard workout. Rushing the rest and repair process can reduce or negate the positive effects of the hard exercise.

Not only do recovery and recuperation give you the ability to regain strength and energy after each workout, but the faster you are able to recover, the faster muscle mass and greater strength will occur.

Here are the fundamentals of creating faster, more complete recoveries to build more muscle mass in a shorter time:

➢ **How fast and how fully** you are able to recover is unique to you and is based on your genetic profile and overall physical condition. The intensity and duration of the calisthenics exercise you performed also determines the recovery time needed. Also, you must consider how much rest time you had *between* each workout.

➢ **How often you exercise** each week is very important. Fewer resistance workouts and more rest time can lead to fuller recovery periods.

➢ **Your diet** plays an influential role, and not just in terms of protein intake. A balanced, healthy diet of diverse, natural, and minimally processed foods (the Mediterranean diet, for example) will supply the vitamins, minerals, antioxidants, and anti-inflammatories needed to optimize the repairs of muscle fibers and cells.

➢ **Stress** can disrupt the rest cycle by activating the sympathetic nervous system's fight-or-flight response and kicking adrenaline and cortisol production into high gear, which elevates heart rate, breathing rate, and blood pressure. It's best to avoid stress always but especially as you recover.

➢ **Rest days** can be any days where you take it easy and are not engaged in high-intensity workouts. Do other things, like hobbies or family time, as opposed to physically challenging activities.

Ideally, you want three workout days per week. At the popular bodybuilding site, Barbell.com, physical trainer Randy Herring (2019), who has over 40 years of conditioning, building solid muscle, and training experience, recommends three good resistance workouts per week. More than three can result in too few rest and recovery periods, and fewer than three may not be enough to achieve the muscular physique you are seeking.

Recuperation time may be divided into three segments:

1. During the workout, take a 30 to 90 second pause between sets (a set is a continuous series of repetitions, or reps, like 15 nonstop push-ups). As you go from exercise to exercise, the 30-90 second pause should be observed, especially if you are repeating sets of the same exercise.
2. Immediately after the exercise is over, take a 2 to 4 hour pause in any other heavy exercise, lifting, climbing stairs, or carrying heavy objects. It's okay to walk and be normally active, however.
3. During the two to three days following exercise, do not perform any resistance exercises, heavy lifting, pulling, or pushing activity. This is the period when the serious rebuilding and recovery takes place, and if you respect this recovery period and limit workouts to three per week, you will be doing the best you can to build lean, large, and well-defined muscles.

The Role of Protein in Recovery

We already know how important nutrition is for building a lean, muscular body, but diet is also an important factor in recovery. The right diet can help replenish energy stores and fluids and optimize the synthesis of protein (a process where amino acids form chains of peptides, which then form complex chains of proteins). Each unit of protein is programmed by our DNA to repair muscles, tendons, ligaments, or any of the trillions of other cells in our bodies. Amino acids and proteins are also essential to building hormones and enzymes. So, if protein is the building block of our muscle cells, fibers, tissues, and organs, having adequate protein in our daily diets is of considerable importance to the recovery process.

Since the damage to muscle cells is actually caused by a depletion of protein, it takes more protein to make the repairs and contribute to the slight overbuilding of the muscle fibers that lead to bigger muscles. And that protein, which contains amino acids, needs to come from our diets. As you learned earlier, you should aim for a 30% caloric intake of lean protein, which can come from plant and animal sources. Having adequate protein available for the recovery also helps prevent the body drawing on healthy protein for repairs (a destructive process called catabolism).

Research published by the International Society of Sports Nutrition (ISSN) shows that athletes following an intense training program can benefit from consuming twice the daily recommended amount of protein or up to 2.0 grams per kg (2.2 lbs). For example, someone who weighs 165 lbs would consume 150 grams of protein per day with or without using a supplement (Kerksick et al., 2018).

Since you will be taking in more than the average amount of daily protein (that 30% of total calories is about 150 grams), it helps to have a protein-rich meal soon after your workout ends. For example, if you workout before breakfast, follow your work out with a breakfast that includes Greek yogurt, two eggs, whole-grain bread, and oatmeal with nuts, flax seeds, and skim milk. You may add meat for added protein but be careful of bacon, which is high in saturated fats, preservatives, and more salt (sodium) than you need. Similarly, if your intense workout is before lunch or dinner, follow with a protein-rich meal afterward.

Should you consider a protein supplement? There are many plant and dairy-based powders and liquids that can provide an average of 15 to 20 grams of protein per serving. According to *Medical News Today,* protein powder may be used to help repair damaged tissues and muscles, and many athletes rely on protein power to accelerate recovery from muscle soreness (Leonard, 2018). Protein supplements taken after intense exercise can speed recovery and improve performance by contributing to muscle protein synthesis (Leonard, 2018).

If amino acid and protein supplements are of interest to you, check the labels for ingredients and try to avoid the brands with a long list of chemical-sounding words. If you're not comfortable with taking supplements, consider getting 18 or 20 grams of natural-sourced protein with a serving of Greek or Icelandic yogurt, which also provides probiotic bacteria that are beneficial to the microbiome in your gut.

Another benefit of a higher-protein diet is weight loss. This is not due to protein being less fattening than carbohydrates, but rather because protein is slower to digest, so it stays in the stomach and gives a feeling of fullness for a longer time. In contrast, carbohydrates and fats are more readily digested, so they pass more quickly through the stomach, leading to hunger pangs.

The Underestimated Importance of Sleep

If we spend eight hours asleep in bed each night, we might think we are wasting valuable time. This attitude encourages many people to sleep fewer hours by staying up late and getting up early. Today's digital age even tempts people to bring their cell phones, tablets, or laptops into the bedroom to keep their days going a little longer.

But it turns out that the traditional advice of "getting a good night's sleep" is medically and scientifically validated. We need eight hours or so, and this is especially true for those, like you, who work out and are trying to build bigger, stronger muscles. Your body needs this full night of restful sleep to rebuild and recover, and so does your brain.

Sleep, it turns out, is as important as intense calisthenics exercise because during sleep, your body initiates the recovery and rebuilding process and gets to work healing the microscopic rips and tears your muscles experienced as you pushed, pulled, and challenged them with hard exercise. The reason for this is that as you sleep, your body is in a high anabolic state, meaning it is better able to fabricate the larger protein molecules that are needed to repair your muscle fibers, your body tissues, your nervous system, and your immune system.

Also, compared to your waking hours when you are active and your muscles are in use, when you are sleeping, your body metabolizes protein more effectively and faster. A full, uninterrupted night of sleep is especially important following an intense workout when cell damage is maximal and protein synthesis is most needed.

When you are asleep, your body is producing testosterone and melatonin, which are human growth hormones crucial for cellular regeneration. The protein production stimulated by these hormones then exceeds protein destruction (because your muscles are inactive), so there is a net gain in muscle fiber size. But upon awakening and throughout the day and evening, protein is being broken down faster than it can be repaired; this is true even on days you do not work out. You probably recognize melatonin for its ability to induce sleep; now, you can appreciate the relationship between melatonin, sleep, and regeneration of muscles.

Physiologist Barry Lumsden (2019), a Level 2 Gym Instructor with 20 years of scientific research supporting his perspectives, recommends a protein-rich beverage before bed on nights following a hard workout. This will ensure that the body's protein stores are not depleted during the night and maximum rebuilding of muscles can occur. Lumsden (2019) suggests that either whey protein or casein protein supplements are excellent for inhibiting protein breakdown during sleeping. Both elevate amino acid levels; however, casein-derived protein tends to last longer.

A further benefit of sleep is stress reduction. Our bodies react to stress by elevating our cortisol hormone levels, which then prompts surges of energy-producing glycogen to the muscles that counter the growth hormone testosterone. It's the familiar fight-or-flight reaction. Stress can be responsible for breaking down muscle tissue and preventing regrowth. A full night's sleep diminishes stress and keeps cortisol levels low and testosterone levels high.

With the need for a full nights' sleep to build muscle and maintain good physical and mental health, how do we establish good sleep habits and stay with them?

Here's how:

1. **Be Consistent** - Go to sleep and wake up at the same time every day. Don't make exceptions on weekends, because the goal is to condition your body to make sleep habitual and regular.
2. **Don't Oversleep** - Oversleeping can reset your internal clock, making it harder to wake up on time the next day. Oversleeping will also make it harder to fall asleep at the prescribed time.
3. **Don't Nap** - Yes, Winston Churchill napped and some people advocate a little siesta after lunch, but naps will leave you less tired at bedtime. A cup of coffee after lunch is a better option.
4. **No Caffeine in the Evening** - It takes four to six hours for the caffeine in your body to diminish sufficiently to not keep you awake. So, that means no caffeine in the evening or before bed.
5. **No Alcohol Before Bedtime** - If you drink (and do so in moderation), do it early enough so that it's out of your system before bedtime. During sleep, alcohol suppresses stage 2 REM

(rapid eye movement) sleep, which is when dreaming occurs and the brain resets itself.

6. **Avoid Sleeping Pills** - Sleeping pills can become a hard-to-break habit, and you don't want to become dependent on them. Like alcohol, some sleeping pills can interfere with dreaming and the resetting of the brain.

7. **No Digital Visitors** - Do not bring your mobile phone, tablet, or laptop into the bedroom. First, whatever you are watching or reading may cause you stress, making it hard for your central nervous system to calm down. Also, the bluish light from these digital screens tend to counter our melatonin production, which normally activates when it is dark. For all these reasons, do not watch television in bed as well.

8. **Keep Your Evenings Calm and Relaxed** - It's best to avoid any stressors before bed. Avoid arguments, confrontations, or emotional talks with family and friends. If you watch TV or stream movies in the evening, steer clear of violent programs, which can raise your pulse rate and breathing rate, simulating the release of cortisol and adrenaline.

9. **Reduce Tension** - If you are feeling tense before bed, take a warm bath or shower. Have a warm beverage, but instead of coffee or tea,

consider warm milk (better than you may think) or hot chocolate.
10. **Make Your Bedroom Conducive To Sleep** - Your sleeping area should be dark and quiet with a good airflow of cool air. If the airflow isn't good, consider a small fan that will also provide a light white noise effect. Keep your bedroom uncluttered so that you don't end up tripping in the dark.

With all the knowledge you have about how to rest and recover correctly, we can now get to the heart of beefy calisthenics and dive into the bodyweight calisthenics exercises and routines you will follow to reach your physical goals, starting with the proper exercise selection.

Chapter 4:

Proper Exercise Selection

Your calisthenics exercise program will be based on the experiences of many different athletes who have experimented and tested, under a wide range of conditions, every type of movement imaginable. Consider the almost infinite number of exercises that are open to you: pushing, pulling, lifting, bending stretching, arching, extending, and compressing among others. Consider how much resistance should be used for each exercise: a lot, a little, or none at all. Consider the element of timing: the speed of performing each movement, the number of repetitions, the number of sets, the time between each set, and the sequence of the exercises. These are all things you will learn to master through the art of proper exercise selection.

Compound vs. Static Exercises

Calisthenics exercises can either involve movement with more than one muscle group working at the same time (compound exercises) or involve no movement with only a single muscle or muscle group working (static exercises). On the whole, compound movements are far better in helping you achieve your fitness goals than static ones.

Compound Exercises

Compound exercises work and challenge multiple muscle groups simultaneously. When you perform a squat, for example, it is a compound exercise that involves working the glutes, the quadriceps, and the calves. A push-up is a compound exercise that engages abdominal muscles, shoulders, triceps quadriceps, and glutes all at the same time. Another type of compound exercise is performing two separate or unrelated exercises at the same time, such as a leg raise while doing lunges. If done by itself, the leg raise would be categorized as an isolation exercise, since it's working only one muscle group (the abdominals). The advantage of compound exercises is working more muscles or muscle groups at the same time, while isolation exercises may be appropriate when a specific muscle needs strengthening, such as during post-injury rehabilitation.

The benefits of compound exercises are based on getting more done in a shorter time, resulting in more muscles worked, more calories burned, better intramuscular coordination, greater strength building, more muscle mass, and increased flexibility. There are cardiovascular benefits, too, since compound exercise raises the heart and breathing rates. Experts consider compound exercises to be the ultimate form of strength training and recommend these multiple exercises to be the central focus of a workout.

Static Exercises

Static exercises, commonly known as isometrics, are distinctly different from compound exercises, as they do not involve movement (that is: there is no shortening or lengthening of the muscles). The muscles are tensed and flexed but are not compressed or expanded. As a result, only moderate amounts of work are being performed, leading to limited improvement in strength and muscle size. While static exercises can work different muscle groups at the same time, they do not challenge the full range of muscular motions and need to be supplemented with the movement of compound exercises.

However, certain static exercises can fit within a bodyweight calisthenics workout; the side plank is a good example of a bodyweight exercise that works multiple muscle groups—abdominals, anterior part of the deltoid, and quadriceps—at the same time. Static exercises can also be used to target the entire body, including challenging several different muscle groups at the same time.

Static exercises are also good for those recovering from injuries or suffering from health conditions who need low-impact exercise. The Mayo Clinic reports that isometric or static exercises may be prescribed to help rehabilitate rotator cuff injuries and arthritis (Salyer, 2016). The online medical journal Healthline.com reports that static (isometric) exercises may be the safer alternative to more strenuous exercise under certain conditions, such as when someone is recovering from knee surgery, a shoulder injury, or a general surgical operation (Salyer, 2016).

Summing up, given your goal of using bodyweight calisthenics to get into great shape and build a physique you are proud of, your workouts should be based primarily (if not exclusively) on compound exercises, rather than relying entirely on single isolation or static isometric exercises.

Whole Body Workout

The best way to achieve a full body workout is to perform a prescribed series of compound exercises, which is known as circuit training, that target the upper body, the core, and the lower body. This way, different muscle groups can be worked sequentially. For example, after doing exercises that challenge your upper body, it is better to move on to the core and then lower body before returning to the upper body again.

You may wonder why a full body workout is necessary. Perhaps, a great set of biceps and shoulders is all you want. Well, first of all, you want to look great from head to toe, but the rationale for a full body workout is about more than aesthetics. You want to have a strong, well-developed body for your health and so that you can tackle all aspects of your life. Further, you want a well-conditioned body that has adequate strength for all types of activities. The major advantage of bodyweight calisthenics over weightlifting is that you avoid overdeveloping certain muscle groups, which means you will have more movement and flexibility.

The following sections describe the nine fundamental bodyweight calisthenics, including the body sections and muscle groups that are worked and how to perform the exercises. In the following chapter, there are further descriptions of the exercises and how to perform them, plus images and links to online videos that demonstrate the movements.

Pull Exercises for Upper Body

Pull exercises develop and train your arms, upper body, back, biceps, and forearms. These pull exercises are very demanding and should be performed two times per week to permit sufficient recovery and rebuilding time.

Pull-Ups

Yes, the pull-ups you may have done in high school are a highly effective exercise for building your upper body. A pull-up is performed by hanging from a bar with your arms shoulder width apart and palms facing forward as you grip the bar. You then pull-up until your head reaches over the bar.

If you have ever found pull-ups tough to do, it's for good reason: A pull-up forces you to lift your entire body weight without assistance. As you think about doing pull-ups, consider the importance of good form. Be more concerned about your technique rather than how many you can perform. You may recall a trainer or coach advising you to go "all the way up and all the way down," and that advice remains solid today. Speed should be moderate, and a slight pause when you reach bottom will prevent a "bounce" back up.

Chin-Ups

These movements appear identical to pull-ups, but the hands are a bit closer together and the palms are facing backward; otherwise, it's the same movement. One key difference in the effect of this movement is the additional work being done by the biceps as well as the shoulders and forearms. As with pull-ups, form is important here. You want a full range of motion: All the way up, head over the bar, all the way down, and not racing through the movements.

Unless you have been doing pull-ups and chin-ups regularly, you will find them tough when first getting started. There is no trick or shortcut; the only way to master these two versions of the pull-up is to do them consistently. You may not be able to do many reps, and that's okay, as long as you do as many as you can and do them correctly. Rest between sets and do the required number of sets. Within a week or two, you will be increasing your reps and after a month, you will be impressed with your progress.

Push Exercises for Upper Body and Core

Push exercises develop and train your arms, chest, triceps, and shoulders, as well as the complexity of central muscles that comprise your core. Push exercises should be performed two or three times per week, depending on intensity, to permit sufficient recovery and rebuilding time.

Push-Ups

Most of us have done push-ups as part of our workouts at some time, but this simple reliable exercise is often overlooked. It deserves our attention and adoption as part of a serious calisthenics workout. Using your bodyweight for resistance, push-ups work, all at the same time, the arms, shoulders, upper body, core, and even lightly the quadriceps. As such, they are an excellent compound exercise. Push-ups super target the chest muscles (pectoral), shoulder muscles (deltoids), upper arms (the triceps), the so-called wing muscles below the armpits (serratus anterior), and the stomach (abdominals).

While there are variations you can try, the basic push-up is a good way to start. Hands are placed shoulder width apart while the back remains straight (no sagging!). You lower your chest to the floor, pause for an instant, and raise up fully on extended arms.

Be less concerned about how many push-ups you can perform during one set; keep the pace slow and the form correct. Push-ups will become easier to perform in greater numbers within a short time.

A challenging variation is to go very slowly, taking 15 or 20 seconds to reach bottom, pause, and then take the same slow time to raise all the way up. Someone who can do 20 or 25 push-ups at normal speed may be challenged to do more than three of these slow versions.

As a starting movement, you can do planks, which are performed by simply assuming the starting push-up position with arms fully extended and back straight. Hold this position for at least 20 seconds, and over time, up to one minute. It gives the core a good workout and prepares the shoulders and arms for later efforts to perform push-ups.

Dips

A dip is a simple movement that helps tighten the core, strengthen the shoulders, and especially works the triceps at the back of your upper arms. Since push-ups also work the same muscle groups, do not perform push-ups and dips in close proximity. Allow some time in-between by doing exercise for the upper body or lower body.

If you have access to parallel bars or any furniture that will allow you to lean forward and lower your upper body, you should be able to perform dips without a problem. But as an alternative, you can do bench dips these two ways:

1. **Option 1**

    Place two benches or chairs parallel to each other and a bit more than your shoulder width apart. Stand between the benches, place your hands on them, and walk your feet forward so that you are in a nearly seated position. Your arms should be fully extended.

Lower your body directly downward, as if you are trying to sit on the floor. You won't reach the floor, but drop down as far as you can, and then rise back up. Perform the planned number of reps, if you can.

2. **Option 2**

Sit on a bench or heavy chair (that will not tip forward) and place your hands on the front edge of the bench or chair wide enough apart to allow room for your body to pass between them.

Slide your bottom forward so you are now suspending your upper body in front of the bench. Lower your body directly downward as far as you can and then rise back up. Perform the planned number of reps or as many as you are able.

However you are able to perform dips, you will be impressed at how well they work the triceps behind your upper arms. If you find your elbows are getting sore, don't descend quite as far during your next set of dips.

Exercises for the Core

The core is the network of interlocking muscles that control and stabilize the body's central torso. It includes the abdominal muscles, the transverse abdominis (technically speaking, the broad and paired muscles on the lateral sides of the abdominal wall), the internal and external abdominal obliques, the erector spinae (a group of muscles and ligaments that straighten and rotate the back), and the right and left lower lats.

Weakness or injury to the core muscles can lead to imbalance, strains, and lower back pain. Further, a weak core will allow abdominal muscles to sag and will result in a protruding waistline and a stooped posture, which is the opposite of what you are hoping to achieve with solid, rippled abs.

Core training exercises can strengthen and develop the core's stabilizing muscles. In addition to the core-strengthening push exercises, like push-ups and dips, there are other exercises that isolate the core muscles, including leg raises, side planks, and Supermans.

Leg Raises

This simple movement is recommended to strengthen the abdominal muscles and the lower back. Leg raises are considered to be more effective and safer than crunches and sit-ups, which may strain lower back muscles. The key to effectively and safely building the abdominal muscles, especially the lower abs, is to perform leg raises slowly and deliberately, being more concerned with form than with how many you can perform in a short time.

To perform leg raises, lie down on your back, either on a mat or carpeted floor (if you have neither a yoga-style foam mat nor carpet, you may spread out a folded blanket so that it's thick and cushioning). Your legs should be extended fully forward. Slide a folded towel under your bottom to raise it slightly. Begin the exercise by raising your head and shoulders a few inches off of the ground. If this feels like it's straining your neck, use your hands to hold your head up.

Now, inhale and raise your legs about 30 degrees or about a foot and a half above the ground. Hold that position for a few seconds and then exhale as you slowly lower your legs. But be sure that they do not touch the ground. Hold them just above the floor. Repeat this cycle for the desired number of reps. If you need to lower your legs all the way to the floor, that's okay; you'll get stronger with time and repetition.

A leg raise variation that can create a compound exercise entails doing leg raises while performing pull-ups or chin-ups. For this, you lift your legs from the vertical position to the horizontal position as you pull yourself up and lower them as you descend. Athletes in top condition can hold their legs in the vertical position throughout the full cycle of reps. An easier version is to lift your knees to your chest as you pull yourself up and then lower the knees as you descend.

Side Planks

This exercise is good for strengthening the core, especially the oblique abdominals, which are not well challenged by crunches or even by leg raises. Side planks also stabilize your hips by strengthening the gluteus maximus and gluteus medius, which are the muscles we sit on! Unlike some other core exercises, side planks do not pressure your neck or lower back, which could lead to strains and injuries. This exercise also helps build balance, leading to ease of movement.

Begin the exercise by lying on your right side with your legs fully extended and the left leg lying directly on top of the right leg (or "stacked") from your thighs to your ankles. Your right elbow should be below your right shoulder. Let your left arm extend along your left side. Pull in your abdominal muscles. Rest your weight on your right elbow and forearm to hold your upper body up. Try to keep your legs and torso aligned and hold the position for as long as you can.

When first starting out, try to hold the side plank for at least 30 seconds. If you feel up to it, raise your left arm and point it to the ceiling. Try not to sag while holding the side plank position. Also, don't roll or fall forward or hold the position for too long. Keep your balance and maintain the correct position. When you feel fatigue or the inability to hold the position, let yourself down carefully. Repeat the exercise lying on your left side.

Depending on your condition, this may be difficult when first starting your bodyweight calisthenics program. If it's too hard to raise up on your right elbow, use your left hand to add to the upward pushing effort. Repeat this two-handed effort on the other side. Other variations to ease into side planks include raising the upper leg (while not trying to push your body up) or lying on an exercise ball. Be patient; this will become easier over time as your balance improves and your strength increases.

Superman

Does "Up, up, and away" come to mind? Can you picture Superman flying through the air with his arms and legs fully extended? That is the position of the Superman pose that you will use to develop your core. This exercise helps build the muscles in the shoulders, the frontal and oblique abdominal groups, and the muscles of your back and legs. The Superman exercise looks easy, but you may find it takes time and practice to master this important movement, which is often adopted by yoga and Pilates practitioners because of its benefits. This exercise both strengthens and increases mobility to help prevent both lower back and upper back injury while giving the entire core, shoulders, and legs a good workout. Sean Alexander, an ACE-certified trainer, says that the Superman is a very effective movement that uses body weight to strengthen the posterior upper and lower back muscles, the abdominals, the glutes, and the hamstrings (which means lower body benefits, too) (Weiner, 2020).

Begin by lying on your stomach on a mat or carpeted surface, not on a hard floor, and extend your legs straight back and your arms fully forward along the sides of your head. Look down, not forward or up. Imagine Superman surveying the ground below and tuck your chin down towards your chest (you'll avoid straining your neck this way). Raise your arms a few inches upwards and, at the same time, raise your legs upwards a few inches as well. Manage the tempo and don't go too fast. Hold the position at the top of each rep for several seconds and then lower your limbs. Pause and repeat.

Here are some suggestions to help performance and create good results:

1. If you find it too hard at first to raise both arms and both legs simultaneously, raise only one arm and one opposite leg at a time (for example, right arm and left leg) and then reverse. You may only be able to lift your limbs slightly, but this will improve.
2. Work on extending the range of motion. Keep breathing slowly and deeply. Do not be tempted to hold your breath. Inhale deeply when you raise your limbs and exhale fully as you lower them.
3. Avoid overextending your arms and limbs, which puts too much strain on them. Instead, maintain a slight bend in your limbs as you perform the exercise.

Lower Body Exercises

The importance of strong legs cannot be overstated. Almost everything we do involves our legs, from walking to running and from climbing to lifting. So, it's good to know that our thigh and calf muscles respond well to bodyweight calisthenics. In fact, as our bodyweight calisthenics program proceeds, they will become bigger, stronger, and more defined.

Squats

This is the definitive bodyweight exercise for the set of quadriceps thigh muscles that extend down the front of our upper legs from hip to knee and for the gluteus maximus, minimus, and medius, better known as the buttock muscles. Squats also work the hamstrings (at the back of the thighs), the adductor groin muscles, the hip flexors, and the calves. Squats are also credited with working the range of core muscles. As these are the largest muscles in our bodies, we burn more calories when we work this group compared to any other.

As important as squats are, they are comparatively easy to perform. You can get through most of the required reps easily with some harder work needed for the last few. But then, you'll feel a rewarding burn or glow when you've stopped.

Begin by standing upright with good posture. Place your hands on opposite shoulders, crossing your arms in front of your chest (this is to help with balance). Your feet should be shoulder width apart, and your weight shifted slightly to your heels.

Now, keeping your back straight, slowly lower downward into a squat position, which is about halfway down. Your thighs should be parallel to the ground, but you have some latitude here. Go down far enough to work the muscles but not so far that your knees begin to hurt (a little crackling of the knees is normal, especially when we mature).

In case you have balance issues and find yourself having to step forward or to the side, simply hold lightly to a chair, table, or counter without using it to relieve any of the weight you are lowering and raising. With practice, you will find it easy to keep from falling over.

Don't lean forward; maintain good posture throughout the movement to ensure keeping your balance. Maintain a slow, consistent pace and don't try to go too fast. Pause when you reach the full squat position, instead of bouncing right back up. Don't hold your breath. Inhale deeply as you squat down. Exhale fully each time you rise back up to the standing position.

Calf Raises

If you have ever seen runners warming up or cooling down by pushing against a tree or a wall, chances are they are stretching their calves. Our calf muscles work hard to propel us forward and help us stand, so they are important to keep strong. The calf raise is one of the easiest exercises to perform, yet it is effective in strengthening and shaping the calf muscles and helping to prevent injury.

Stand with feet close together or slightly apart with weight distributed evenly. Rise up on the balls of your feet and your toes by raising your heels. Stand upright, and you should be able to perform calf raises without holding on for balance. But if you need a little assistance, lightly hold on to a table or chair. Rise fully, pause, and lower for the prescribed number of reps.

For increased extension and compression of the calf muscles, stand with the front part of your feet on a stair, a book, or anything that keeps the heels lower than the toes. When you rise, a greater effort is required to achieve the longer range of motion.

Another calf raise variation is to bend your knees slightly as you perform the raising and lowering. This shifts the workload to the soleus muscle, which is smaller but equal in importance to the larger gastrocnemius muscle (the one we see as the major calf muscle).

With this orientation to proper exercise selection now completed, we are ready to move to the specific details that will more completely familiarize you with these nine fundamental exercises and enable you to perform them with confidence.

Chapter 5:

Nine Fundamental Movements to Master

Now that you have become familiar with compound exercises and the fundamental bodyweight calisthenic movements, you are ready to master these nine exercises and build a solid foundation that will fulfill your expectations of achieving a strong, muscular body that you can be proud of.

Each of these nine calisthenics exercises was reviewed in detail in the previous chapter; however, here, they are presented in a streamlined format with images and videos so that you can start practicing them quickly and correctly.

> ➤ Take advantage of the links provided that lead to online demonstrations of the exercises, positions, and movements. You may click on the link in the *How* section to start each brief *YouTube.com* video presentation. (You will see a brief commercial when most of the videos

begin; look for the small "Skip Ads" button on the lower right to begin the demo.)

Pull-Ups

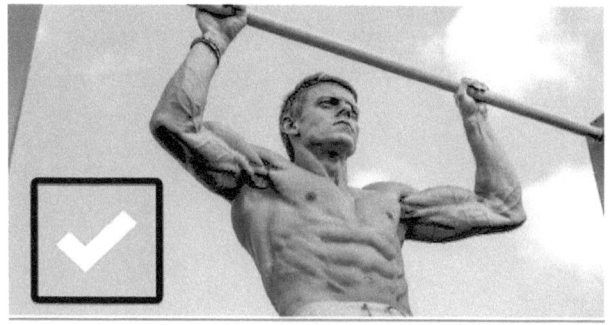

Fig. 2

Where: You will need a horizontal bar that is at the height of your extended arms, and if there is nothing available at home, you can usually find a bar to use in a park or recreation area. There are pull-ups/chin-up bars that can be purchased, too (this is the only equipment you might need to buy for this complete workout).

How: Reach up to grasp the bar with both hands, palms forward. Your arms should be shoulder width apart. Pull slowly up until your head is above the bar. Pause for a split second and then lower back down. Extend fully. Repeat the pull-up cycle up to the plan limit or as many as you can without jerking, kicking your legs, or failing to reach the bar.

Link to the video demo: https://www.youtube.com/watch?v=eGo4IYlbE5g

Result: This is primarily an upper-body exercise. You will feel the effort in your upper arms, lower arms, and especially the shoulders. There is usually some additional work performed by the core muscles, such as the back and the abdominals, if the legs are engaged by pulling or raising them up during the pull-up cycle.

Chin-Ups

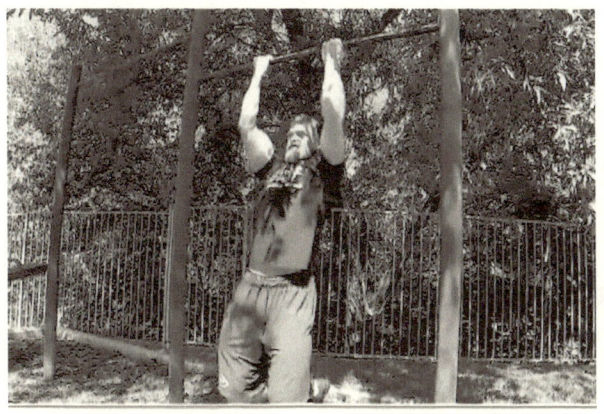

Fig. 3

Where: The chin-up is the fraternal twin of the pull-up and is performed under the same "where/what" conditions with a horizontal bar that is at least arm-reach height.

How: The movement is the same as pull-ups with the exception of the grip: The backs of the hands are placed face forward and the palms and fingertips are facing toward you. The hands may be placed closer to each other than shoulder width. As with pull-ups, the movements should be slow and steady without jerking. Try to fully reach the bar with your head (ideally, your chin) and fully extend at the bottom.

Link to the video demo: https://www.youtube.com/watch?v=brhRXlOhsAM

Result: Compared to pull-ups, there will be more work done by the biceps with chin-ups, and you may feel a warm glow and heat (due to blood and hormones accumulating) as the bicep is being pumped up. Shoulders, lower arms, and core muscles will also be worked.

Push-Ups

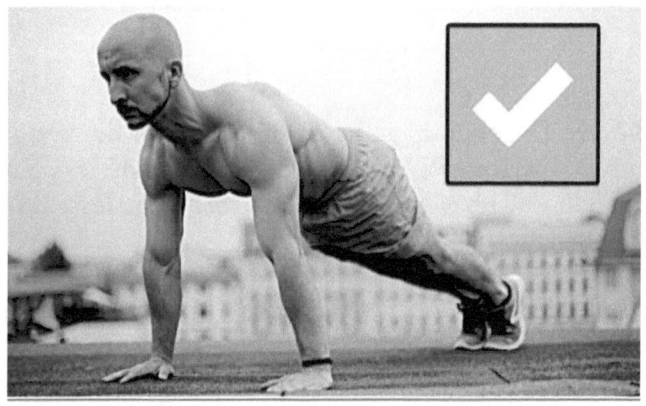

Fig. 1

Where: Perform push-ups on any flat surface.

How: Begin with your legs fully extended behind you and your body supported by your fully extended arms.

Your hands should be under your shoulders so that hands, elbows, and shoulders are in a straight vertical line. Slowly, lower your chest to the floor, keeping your back straight (no sagging!). Push back up to the beginning position, remembering to keep your back straight. Repeat for the planned number of reps and sets. Don't bounce right back up when you've fully lowered, but there's no need to pause, either. If you're finding it tough when starting out and want to make your push-ups easier, drop down on both knees. To make push-ups more challenging, slow the pace down, taking longer to lower and raise.

Link to the video demo:
https://www.youtube.com/watch?v=IODxDxX7oi4&feature=youtu.be

Result: This classic compound exercise is great for building up your core strength as well as challenging and building strong shoulders.

Dips

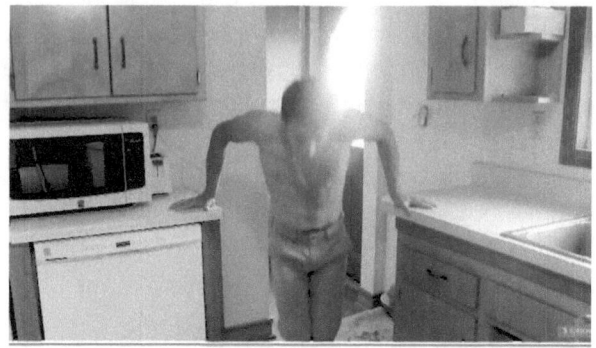

Fig. 5

Where: Dips can be performed at home using chairs, boxes, benches, or countertops, as shown above. Just be sure that whatever you will be dipping with is steady and won't easily tip as you lower yourself.

How: Place your hands on the two separate surfaces so that you can lower yourself between them. Lift your feet and cross your ankles. Slowly, lower yourself as far as possible without straining and then push yourself back up to complete one rep. An alternative form of a dip is to lower yourself on a single chair, bench, or countertop. To do this, grasp the edge of the surface and extend your legs forward. While holding your weight with the palms of both hands, slide your body forward far enough so that your bottom can pass in front of the surface. Lower your body by bending your elbows, going as low as you can without straining and push back up. Repeat as specified in the plan. To make it easier, slide your feet back so that your knees are bent.

Link to the video demo: https://www.youtube.com/watch?v=isikOOF0W3k

Result: You will feel the workout mostly in your triceps (the back of your arms), plus your shoulders.

Leg Raises

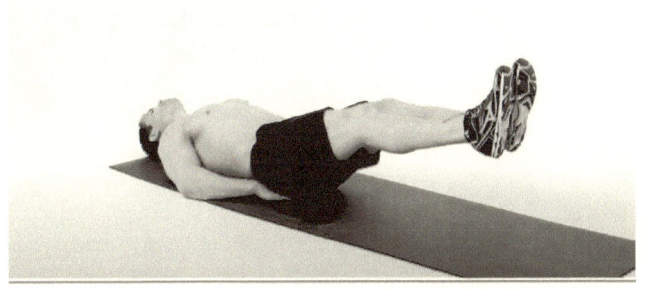

Fig. 6

Where: On the floor with a yoga mat (or any foam mat) or carpet (a folded blanket should work well, too).

How: Lie on your back with your legs fully extended. Place a folded towel under your hips so they are slightly elevated (or you may slide your hands under you to lift your hips, as seen above). The movement begins by raising your heels about 18 inches off of the floor. You should feel a slight tensing of the abdominal muscles. Now, raise your legs all the way up so that they point at the ceiling and pause. Slowly, lower to the starting position. Keep your heels from touching the ground and raise the legs for each of the reps in the set. Try to keep your legs straight throughout the movement, but if you're finding it hard, bend your knees. As mentioned previously, you can make this a compound exercise by performing leg raises while doing pull-ups or chin-ups.

Link to the video demo: https://www.youtube.com/watch?v=l4kQd9eWclE

Result: Leg raises are great for the core, including the frontal abdominal muscles, the lower abs, and the lower back muscles. If you find your neck has become sore, place a small folded towel under your head to avoid the strain.

Side Planks

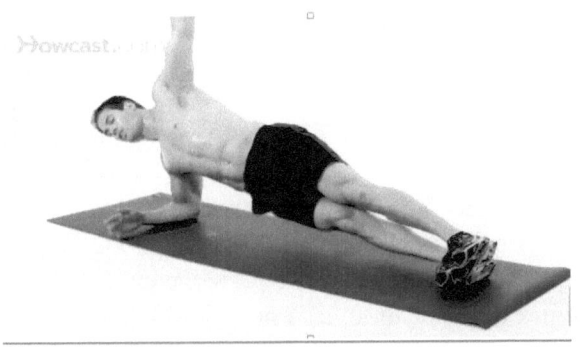

Fig. 7

Where: On the floor with a foam mat, carpet, or a folded blanket for support.

How: Roll over onto your right side, extend your legs fully, and place your left leg on top of the right leg. Rest your upper body weight on your right forearm and right elbow, which should be directly under the right shoulder. Place your left hand on your left hip. Now, push your hips upwards, supporting your body with the right elbow and forearm. Align your legs and body in a straight line. One option is to raise your left arm and point it toward the ceiling. You may find this movement difficult when first starting out, so you can use your left hand to press down on the floor, which will assist considerably in getting your hips up in the air. You may also find it easier if your left leg remains on the floor in front of your right leg. Do your best to raise your hips even a little, knowing you will get stronger with practice. Hold the side plank position for up to 30 seconds starting out (you'll do it longer as you develop). Once you complete the side plank on the right side, roll over and repeat on the left side.

Link to the video demo: https://www.youtube.com/watch?v=NXr4Fw8q60o

Results: Once you are able to perform this movement even partially, you will be improving your core, the oblique abdominals, and the glutes, which stabilize the hips and improve balance. Your shoulders will get some work, too.

Superman

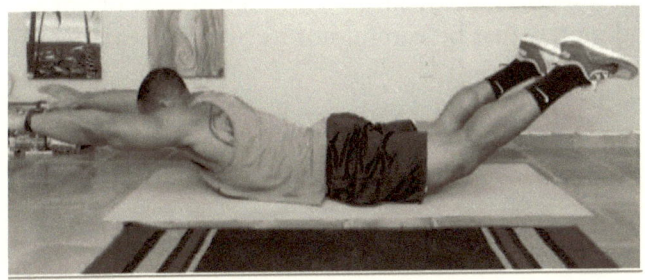

Fig. 8

Where: On the floor, supported by a foam mat, carpet, or folded blanket. Allow enough room so that you can fully extend your arms and legs.

How: Reach as far forward as you can with arms against your head and legs stretched behind you with toes extended back. Raise your hands and arms a few inches. Do the same with your legs. Ideally (and this may take some time and practice), the arms will be raised from your shoulders and your legs will be raised from your hips. An interim version to build strength is to raise one arm and the opposing leg and then reversing the sequence (right arm and left leg and then left arm and right leg). Keep the emphasis on raising the arms and legs and not arching the lower back.

Link to the video demo: https://www.youtube.com/watch?v=VUT1RHyMEuc

Results: This is one of the finest exercises to develop the core, including the front abdominals and upper and lower back. It also benefits your upper arms, shoulders, and the lower body, such as the hamstrings, hip flexors, and glutes. Just be careful not to over flex or strain the lower back.

Squats

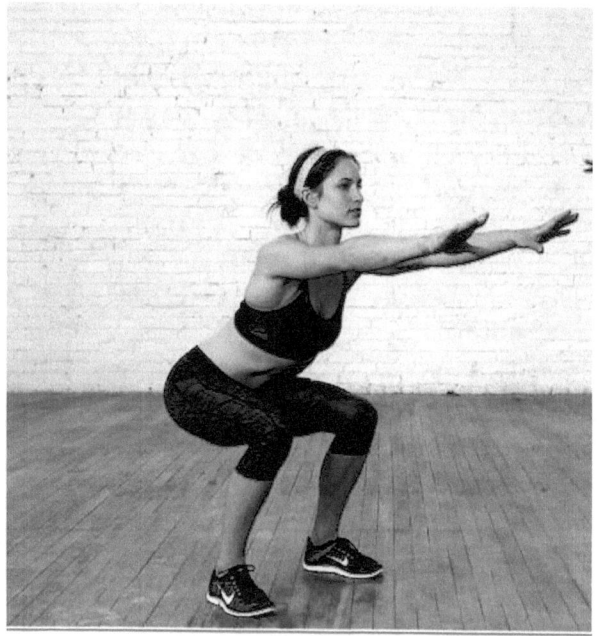

Fig. 9

Where: Any flat, hard surface. A chair or table is optional for assisting with balance. Also, you can perform the movement with a wall close behind as to prevent accidentally falling backward.

How: Stand upright with your feet shoulder width apart and with your weight shifted slightly back toward your heels. Angle your toes outward. Keeping your back straight, bend your knees and squat as if sitting down in a chair. Keep your knees pointing forward. If done correctly, your knees will remain over your toes and should not extend past them. To keep your balance, you may extend your arms forward, or if balance is still challenging, place the fingers of one hand on a nearby chair, table, or counter. Don't place any weight on it; it's just to steady yourself. Try to lower until your thighs are parallel to the floor. Keep alert to maintain upright posture throughout the movement. Rise from the squat with the same good form and repeat the required reps.

Link to the video demo: https://www.youtube.com/watch?v=aclHkVaku9U

Result: A well-performed set of squats will be felt warmly in the quadriceps at the front of your thighs. They will also tone your hamstrings, calves, and hip flexors.

Calf Raises

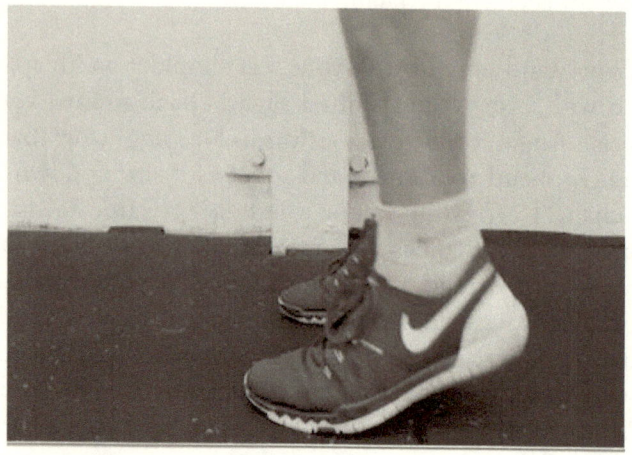

Fig. 10

Where: Any flat, hard surface or on a step, if a longer movement is desired. A chair or table is optional for assisting with balance. This exercise may also be performed by standing on a flat surface that is 1-2 feet from a wall, tree, or pole.

How: It's as simple as raising up on the balls of the feet and toes, pausing, and lowering to the floor. At the top of the raise, you will feel the muscles of your calf compressing. If you are standing on a step with your heels extended, lower all the way down so your heels are well below the level of the step and your toes. An easier version of calf raises is to perform them while seated in a chair.

Link to the video demo: https://www.youtube.com/watch?v=TZrBb5M1CdM

Result: While calf raises are easy to do, at the end of the set, your calves should feel good (no pain) with a warm sense of exertion.

Now, it's time to develop your personal workout plan, which is a schedule that takes into account your level of conditioning and establishes how the next three weeks will unfold. Each of the nine bodyweight calisthenic exercises will be scheduled with sequences per day, repetitions, and sets. You will do exercises most days of the week, because you will be rotating different muscle groups. So, while one group rests, another gets to work. The important rest periods are included but don't expect time off. Calisthenics are a daily commitment, but as indicated, hard workouts will be separated by two or three recovery days.

Chapter 6:

Your 21-Day Workout Plans

We have so far provided you with the foundation of how to build muscles and get fit and stronger with bodyweight calisthenics. The next step is learning how to schedule your workouts so that each day you know *what* to do and *how* to do it. Here, you will explore two 21-day plans that will get you going right away and keep you going over the long haul. In addition, your planning will integrate two other key elements of your conditioning: cardiovascular exercise and a healthy, protein-rich diet.

The Importance of Planning

Extensive experience has convinced generations of trainers and physical therapists that planning plays a decisive role in determining how effectively an individual will train and achieve their fitness and strength goals. If you have been to a gym or fitness center, you have probably seen trainers working with their clients by following a prescribed schedule of exercise movements, day by day, week by week, and month by month. When it's done right, planning ensures steady progress without imposing excessive strain or causing injuries. In fact, many coaches believe that overdoing workouts and pushing and pulling too much, too fast leads to burnout, strains, or pulls that can set back bodyweight training programs by weeks or months.

To achieve the muscular body you desire, while avoiding injury and overwork, trust the plans that you will be following here. They have been designed with your success and well-being in mind. Even though you will not be using weights and resistance machines, do not underestimate the benefits of using your own bodyweight to perform each exercise. Yes, bodyweight calisthenics are safer than dumbbells, barbells, cables, and machines. When done correctly in the right form with the prescribed reps, sets, rotations, and resting phases, you will build bigger, well-defined muscles with distinctive "cut" musculature. You will also become stronger and faster than you could imagine.

Cardio Exercise and Diet Plan

Your bodybuilding plan would not be complete without the two additional elements of cardiovascular conditioning and a responsible, nutritious diet. There is a strong medically proven basis for performing cardiovascular exercises that systematically raise your pulse rate and breathing rate for a sustained period. These exercises can be performed at least several times a week and in a variety of ways, such as walking, hiking fast, jogging, running, swimming, biking, and using an elliptical machine among the more popular options. Cardiovascular training is important for your overall conditioning and health and will be included in your planning,

If you did not spend too much time digesting (pardon the pun) chapter 2's discussion of nutrition, make sure you give it a second look and also review the role of protein in your diet to optimize muscle building that's covered in chapter 3. Eating a great healthy diet will support and enhance the results of your training. Or, you can ignore good dietary practices, which can slow your bodybuilding results and risk your health.

By including the life-enhancing benefits of bodyweight calisthenics resistance exercises, regular cardiovascular conditioning, and a healthy diet, you will not only be achieving your primary goals of looking good, feeling good, and getting much stronger but you will also be making yourself more resistant to obesity, diabetes, heart disease, and even cancer. Regular intensive resistance and cardiovascular exercise along with a Mediterranean (or similar) diet can reduce or eliminate stress, anxiety, inflammation, and depression. There are encouraging findings that these combined disciplines can slow or stop the onset of dementia, Alzheimer's disease, and Parkinson's, among other degenerative disorders as well.

Taken in the holistic sense, your adoption of and commitment to a comprehensive exercise and diet plan is the most important investment you can make.

A Note of Caution

The UK's respected School of Calisthenics has built their training programs around the concept of hypertrophy, which you may recall refers to building the skeletal muscle fibers by working them hard so they are damaged and need to be rebuilt by the protein in our bodies ("Bodyweight training and workouts," 2020). This healthy damage is caused by forceful tension, which, of course, we supply through resistance exercises. The levels of resistance must be sufficient to truly work the mussels hard, yet not so forceful or long-lasting as to cause serious damage, such as tears, strains, and pulls. That brings us to some practical words of caution to help prevent injuries that can sideline you and your bodybuilding schedule.

It's important to listen to your body, not too closely, or you may overreact. But generally, pain is a warning that should not be ignored. With experience, you will learn to recognize the difference between the normal feeling of exhaustion, like a burn, when you are nearing the end of a set and you're pushing out a few more reps and the real pain that signals that serious damage is being done.

One of the important advantages of bodyweight calisthenics training is that there are limits to the weight you are lifting; you increase the workload mostly by increasing reps and sets, and not by adding 20 lb weights to a barbell, for example.

Shoulders

One well-known area of injury from resistance exercises (or any heavy lifting) are the shoulders. The group of muscles that control shoulder movements are known as the rotator cuff, and once you've done hard damage here, you can be in for a long rehabilitation. Be especially careful not to push your shoulders beyond their limit. Pay attention to any warning signs or extreme pain and ratchet back the tension when it starts to really hurt.

Exercises to watch out for when it comes to possible shoulder injuries are pull-ups, chin-ups, and push-ups, which nonetheless are great for building your shoulders. Also, when performing side planks, your shoulder will be working hard, especially as you push your hips off the floor to rise to the holding position, so pay close attention here as well.

Another cause of rotator cuff injury is not from damage caused by pulling or lifting too much weight but from excessive or repetitive use. You may be aware of baseball pitchers being sidelined for extended rehabilitation exercises or, worse, rotator cuff surgery. Consider that pitching seven innings can involve seven sets of 24 reps (or more) of maximum exertion (throwing the ball at 90 miles per hour with additional arm and shoulder twists to create curves and screwballs). Your 21-day plans will take into account the need to avoid excessive repetition of certain muscle groups.

Lower Back

The lower back, or lumbar region of the spine, is another area of your body that is susceptible to strain and injury. Avoid arching your back during calisthenic movements. For example, don't let your back sag during push-ups; instead, keep your back straight throughout the pushing up and down and during the pause at the top of the movement.

Be careful, too, when performing the Superman exercise, because it does involve a slight arching of the back. Keep the emphasis on raising arms, shoulders, and legs while keeping lower back arching to a minimum. When doing leg raises, be sure to place a folded towel or your hands under your butt to take the strain off the lower back.

Knees

Your knees are a complicated assembly of muscles, tendons, ligaments, and, of course, your kneecaps. Your quadriceps muscle helps hold the kneecap in place as it swivels and adjusts to everything from walking to squatting. The knee is susceptible to *pattern overload repeat injury,* including torn muscles, pulled ligaments, and the erosion of the lubricating cartilage under the kneecap (ask a marathon runner about "runner's knee" symptoms).

The one exercise of the nine you'll be starting with that could aggravate or injure your knees are squats. Do not squat deeper than is comfortable, and do not let your knees extend forward past your toes.

But generally, if you follow the gradual building up of resistance and increased repetitions that your 21-day plans will prescribe, you should build muscle bulk and strength gradually and safely. Resistance training, when done correctly, can create the right conditions for muscle building adaptations to take place in the body as you pressure the muscles to overcome the resistance, force, and the new stress being applied.

Positivity and Motivation

Your attitude is as important as the exercises you will be performing. Having the goal of a stronger, more muscular body and a healthier, more robust persona is the starting point. Yet, the next step is having the self-discipline and tenacity to achieve and sustain your goals.

To sum it up succinctly: "Ya gotta believe," as New York Mets player Tug McGraw famously exhorted his teammates when trying to boost their confidence so that they could make it to the World Series (yes, they made it). You need to believe that your bodyweight calisthenics training program is working, building strength, and adding bulk at the molecular and muscular fiber level every day. And that it is happening as a direct result of the time and effort you put into faithfully and correctly performing the exercises.

Experience shows that, for most people, it's hard to start a fitness program, whether it's calisthenics, traditional resistance with weights, or a cardiovascular routine. Experience also shows that starting the program does not ensure continuing with it. How many people do we know who joined a fitness center only to show up once or twice and then stop? You know the excuses, the most common being, "I don't have the time." Really? Someone who wants to get into shape doesn't have 30 to 45 minutes to spare? It's hard to believe that the great feeling of a workout and the benefits of building muscle and getting stronger are not worth that little bit of time.

No, it's not about time; it's about motivation. People who aspire to shape up, get strong, and get fit but don't commit to the routine just don't have the resolve to get started or to keep it going.

How can you ensure that you are motivated to become an acolyte of bodybuilding and overall physical fitness? How can you be confident you will follow the 21-day plans that will get you started easily and take you gradually to higher and higher levels of strength and musculature?

It goes back to "Ya gotta believe." You need to believe deeply that this really works, and you will get out of it exactly what you put into it.

Have you heard of *The Power of Positive Thinking*? It became a bestselling book when Dr. Norman Vincent Peale published it back in the 1950s, and it still influences millions around the world. The concept is simple and applicable to your fitness goals.

You must:

1. **Visualize yourself succeeding.** See yourself with the physique you aspire to and make it a reality in your mind. Imagine yourself performing each bodyweight calisthenics exercise and feel your muscles bulging and firming.
2. **Think positively** about who you are and what you can do. Tell yourself repeatedly that you are on your way to the musculature you dream of. Do not allow negative thoughts or fear of failure affect you.
3. **Minimize any obstacles** that might interfere with your scheduled exercises. Treat your workout time as sacrosanct, inviolable, and untouchable. Dismiss possible obstacles in your workout with the positive affirmation of "I've got this."

Pre-Planning Principles

While the fundamentals of bodybuilding are similar between bodyweight calisthenics and weightlifting, there is a big difference when it comes to increasing the tension so that you can progress to challenging the muscles more. With weightlifting, you simply increase the amount of weight being lifted. There's no need to change the numbers of reps or sets, change the timing of the movements, or change the rest and recovery times. But with calisthenics, your weight remains about the same. So with a pull-up, for example, you can only pull-up your weight, no more and no less. The same goes for chin-ups, push-ups, dips, squats, and calf raises. If you weigh 165 lbs, you can only pull or push 165 lbs.

Therefore, different variables need to come into play to increase the challenge to the muscles when you are doing bodyweight calisthenics. Just as weights can be added to increase resistance, with calisthenics we can adjust the exercise movements in terms of positions, angles, and range of motions to work the muscles harder.

First, just to be clear on the terminology:

1. A **rep** (repetition) is one full cycle of an exercise. For instance, the one up-and-down movement of a push-up. To start, you'll probably be doing six to 12 reps for most of the exercises.
2. A **set** is the group of reps you perform in one sequence. So, your six reps of push-ups, for example, make one set of push-ups. You'll be doing about three to five sets at first.

3. **Rest** refers to the interval between sets, which is 30 to 90 seconds.
4. **Recovery** means the number of days between workouts for a body group. For example, recovering for two days between upper body exercises and working out different body groups during those two days.

Okay, here's what you can do to raise the intensity and muscular stress of the exercises without changing your own weight:

1. You can **increase** the numbers of reps and number of sets. For example, increasing from six to 10 reps to 12 reps. Or, increasing from three to five sets to six sets.
2. You can **shorten** the rest time between sets. For example, instead of a 90-second rest, you take a 60- or 30-second rest.
3. You can perform the movements **more slowly,** which increases the tension. For example, when performing push-ups, taking ten seconds to lower and ten seconds to push back up (try it; it's impressive).

You can also add in some of the variants we discussed earlier. For example, as you advance, you can make a push-up more difficult by placing your hands closer together or very far apart. You could also alter the body angle to perform a pike push-up, which increases the intensity and tension on the shoulders and upper chest. Or, there the more challenging archer pull-ups, Korean dips, one-arm push-ups, and one-arm pull-ups. You will have the option in the advanced plan to try these or stick with the more basic exercises where you increase reps and sets while slowing the movements.

There is also the option of adding weight to your body. For example, wearing a weighted vest to add 20 pounds while you are doing push-ups, pull-ups, chin-ups, and most of the other exercises. This is an accepted practice among some calisthenics enthusiasts, but to others, it violates the principle of using only your own bodyweight for resistance.

The one variable you will *not be changing* is the recovery period. A full two days (in most cases) is required so that the necessary protein-based repairs to muscles can be made. This is especially needed as the movements become more challenging.

Your objective is to build tension throughout all of the muscles of your body, integrating many different body parts during the bodyweight-challenging movements. This is why calisthenics are more beneficial than the more isolated movements performed with weights and the pushing and pulling of machine training.

Beginning with the Basics

Each of the 21-day plans will be working the three main muscle groups: the upper body (the arms and the shoulders), the core (the abdominals, back muscles, and side muscles), and the lower body (the quadriceps, the hamstrings, the calves, and the hip flexors). The plans include the nine exercises that you have become familiar with, and each can be modified as you progress with variations in form, procedure, and timing.

The order of each exercise within your plan is based on spacing out similar muscle groups. You wouldn't want to immediately follow three sets of pull-ups with three sets of chin-ups or follow squats with leg raises. However, you are free to vary the order to suit your preferences, as long as you perform the recommended number of reps and sets for the specified cycle times.

You may conduct your bodyweight calisthenics workout sessions two or three days per week or more often, such as five or six days per week. The difference between these two extremes is important.

1. **Two or three** bodyweight calisthenics workouts per week means you will perform all nine exercises for the required reps, sets, cycle times, and set intervals just two or three days per week. In other words, you will have fewer workout training sessions but they will be longer, more intensive workouts. The two or three workouts per week total seven intense workout days during the 21-day schedule.

2. **Four or five** workout days per week may be preferred by those who like almost daily calisthenics sessions. For that option, the plan alternates between two exercise groups: Group 1 with five exercises and Group 2 with four exercises. This option results in four or five calisthenics workouts per week or 14 workout days during the 21-day schedule.

21-Day Plan: Four or Five Exercises Per Session

This 21-day plan divides the nine exercises into two groups of four or five exercises per session.

Movement	Muscle Groups	Reps	Sets	Cycle Time *	Between Sets	21-Day Schedule
Group 1						
Pull-Ups	Upper Body	6	3	3-4 seconds	90 seconds	1 - 4 - 7 - 10 - 13 - 16 - 19
Leg Raises	Core Lower Body	6	3	5 seconds	90 seconds	1 - 4 - 7 - 10 - 13 - 16 - 19
Superman	Core Upper Body Lower	6	3	3 seconds	60 seconds	1 - 4 - 7 - 10 - 13 - 16 -

	Body					19
Dips	Upper Body	6	3	4 seconds	90 seconds	1 - 4 - 7 - 10 - 13 - 16 - 19
Squats	Lower Body	6	3	4 seconds	60 seconds	1 - 4 - 7 - 10 - 13 - 16 - 19
Group 2						
Push-Ups	Upper Body Core	8	3	4 seconds	90 seconds	3 - 6 - 9 - 12 - 15 - 18 - 21
Calf Raises	Lower Body	14	3	8 seconds	30 seconds	3 - 6 - 9 - 12 - 15 - 18 - 21
Side Planks	Upper Body Core	1 each side	3	30 seconds	90 seconds	3 - 6 - 9 - 12 - 15 - 18 -

						21
Chin-Ups	Upper Body	6	3	3-4 seconds	90 seconds	3 - 6 - 9 - 12 - 15 - 18 - 21

*One cycle is the time it takes to complete the movement in seconds. For example, one pull-up cycle includes the pulling up and lowering down movement, while one Superman cycle includes holding the position.

The below chart shows how the two groups will be performed over the 21-day schedule. This plan provides 14 workout days and seven rest/recovery days. The groups are performed on consecutive days, followed by one rest/recovery day, which means each group is separated by two days.

Day/Action	Mon	Tue	Wed	Thu	Fri	Sat	Sun
Days 1 to 7	1	2	3	4	5	6	7
Action	Group 1	Rest	Group 2	Group 1	Rest	Group 2	Group 1
Days 8 to 14	8	9	10	11	12	13	14

Action	Rest	Group 2	Group 1	Rest	Group 2	Group 1	Rest
Days 15 to 21	15	16	17	18	19	20	21
Action	Group 2	Group 1	Rest	Group 2	Group 1	Rest	Group 2

21-Day Plan: Nine Exercises Per Session

This is the one-day-on/two-days-off pattern with all nine exercises performed during one session.

Movement	Muscle Groups	Reps	Sets	Cycle Time	Between Sets	21-Day Schedule
Pull-Ups	Upper Body	6	3	3-4 seconds	90 seconds	1 - 4 - 7 - 10 - 13 - 16 - 19

Exercise	Body Area	Reps	Sets	Tempo	Rest	Weeks
Leg Raises	Core, Lower Body	6	3	5 seconds	90 seconds	1 - 4 - 7 - 10 - 13 - 16 - 19
Superman	Core, Upper Body, Lower Body	6	3	3 seconds	60 seconds	1 - 4 - 7 - 10 - 13 - 16 - 19
Dips	Upper Body	6	3	4 seconds	90 seconds	1 - 4 - 7 - 10 - 13 - 16 - 19
Squats	Lower Body	6	3	4 seconds	60 seconds	1 - 4 - 7 - 10 - 13 - 16 - 19
Push-Ups	Upper Body, Core	8	3	4 seconds	90 seconds	1 - 4 - 7 - 10 - 13 - 16 - 19
Calf Raises	Lower Body	14	3	8 seco	30 second	1 - 4 - 7 -

				nds	s	10 - 13 - 16 - 19
Side Planks	Upper Body Core	1 each side	3	30 seconds	90 seconds	1 - 4 - 7 - 10 - 13 - 16 - 19
Chin-Ups	Upper Body	6	3	3-4 seconds	90 seconds	1 - 4 - 7 - 10 - 13 - 16 - 19

The below chart shows how the nine exercises will be performed over the 21-day schedule. As noted, this plan provides seven workout days and 14 rest/recovery days during the 21-day schedule.

Day	Mon	Tue	Wed	Thu	Fri	Sat	Sun
1 to 7	1	2	3	4	5	6	7
Action	All 9	Rest	Rest	All 9	Rest	Rest	All 9
8 to	8	9	10	11	12	13	14

14							
Action	Rest	Rest	All 9	Rest	Rest	All 9	Rest
15 to 21	15	16	17	18	19	20	21
Action	Rest	All 9	Rest	Rest	All 9	Rest	Rest

Your Initial Progress

You are now ready to get started. Your first decision should be whether you prefer the plan with four to five workouts per week or the alternative of limiting the number of days you exercise. You certainly have the option of trying each schedule to see how they work or don't work for you. Be sure you are getting sufficient rest and recovery between workouts no matter which plan you choose.

Next, you should try to follow the recommended reps, sets, and timing. But since no two of us are equal, you might find *fewer is better* for you in the early days of your training. Or, you may find that you can easily do more. If you can do more reps at a slower pace, with shorter rests between sets, and without strain, by all means, push yourself forward.

As for your initial progress, you're starting on an ambitious bodyweight calisthenics program with high expectations and are hoping you won't be disappointed. Don't worry, you won't be let down. That is, as long as you remember the importance of commitment and dedicate yourself to your bodybuilding goals.

To ensure that you stick with your plan, first and foremost, make some decisions that will ease into your workouts and keep them going on schedule for the first 21-day plan.

Here are some key issues to consider as you embark on your chosen 21-day plan:

1. **Where?**

    Ideally, the best location for your exercise routine is a room or place in your home that has the space you need and the features or fixtures that can be of help.

    Consider: Does the room have carpeting that will cushion you during Superman, and leg raises, and side planks? If not, do you have a yoga mat or a blanket you can fold into a cushion? What about privacy? It's better to avoid distractions so you can focus on your movements and feel your muscles working. You may be more comfortable not having others watch your workout or make comments.

While your home may have the space you need, it may be necessary to go elsewhere to find a bar for pull-ups and chin-ups; although, it would be great to have your own chinning bar. One of these will be safe to use, and most models can be put up and taken down quickly so you can avoid trouble with roommates, friends, spouses, and partners. There are lots of chinning bar options available online. Search the keywords "chinning bar doorway" on Google or [click on this link for a directory](#).

You're not limited to your home; a nearby playground or park may have a bar or equipment, like monkey bars, that you can use. Same goes for structures that you can use for dip exercises.

2. **When?**

The time of day and the days you select to exercise can have a very strong influence, positively or negatively, on whether you stick with your bodybuilding calisthenics program or not. Think through the issue of timing and then be decisive. You need to select one time of day and stick with it.

For example, it's best to work out early morning and before breakfast or, if your schedule allows it, before lunch. If you are a slow starter and pre-breakfast or pre-lunch workouts won't work for you, try before dinner. But don't workout out late, before bed, or after a meal.

Whatever time works for you, commit to it. It will be a mistake to tell yourself you'll work out early in the day, for example, and then decide you'll "get to it later." Chances are, you won't. Consistency and commitment are essential components of achieving your fitness goals.

The same goes for the days you select to exercise. The 21-day schedules can start on any day (no need to wait for Monday), but once you start, it's important to respect the "on" workout days and the "off" rest and recovery days. Of course, things can come up, but if you miss a day, get back to the schedule the next day. As we've emphasized, rest is very important, so an extra recovery day is okay, but don't let it turn into a series of missed days or the progress you've made can start to diminish.

3. **Being Inclusive**

The nine exercises that will be your initial routine have been selected with careful consideration to ensure that your entire body will be challenged, developed, and built-up, so it is important to perform all of these exercises, not just some.

Do not be tempted to concentrate exclusively on your upper body, for example, so you just have impressive biceps, triceps, and shoulders. Give your entire core your equal attention; the same goes for the lower body.

There is a synergistic effect when all nine exercises are performed with equal attention, because your muscles form an interactive network. Every exercise affects multiple regions and muscle groups. Your pull-ups and chin-ups may be very focused on arms and shoulders, but there are tensions extending through your chest, abdominals, and upper back, for example.

4. **Form and Intensity**

Be sure to follow the instructions provided in chapters 4 and 5 about how to perform the nine exercises. These instructions were developed with the objective of helping you perform them fully and correctly. Also, be sure to watch the demo videos. Further, feel free to do your own research, since there are many other demonstrations that you can find online (although, what has been provided here is comprehensive and complete).

You want to perform each exercise correctly and fully; no cheating or shortcuts. When doing push-ups, it's all the way down and all the way back up with a straight back and a momentary pause at the top and bottom positions. You want to ensure you are doing it right. The same goes for pull-ups and push-ups. Half measures will reduce the effectiveness of the movement and diminish the muscle-building effects.

No racing through it, either. Watch your speed and do the movements slower rather than faster, which will ensure the correct amount of tension is being experienced. As you progress in the coming weeks and months, slowing down the movements will be one of the more effective ways to make the exercises more challenging without having to add extra weight. But even at the beginning levels, take it easy.

Feel the tension as you lower and raise back up, pull up and lower down, or sink into each squat. By going slowly, you should be assured that your muscles are receiving sufficient intensity to experience hypertrophy.

Cardiovascular Conditioning

Raising your heartbeat and keeping it elevated for a sustained period is the fundamental objective of aerobics, or cardiovascular conditioning. You're certainly aware of it, seeing joggers everywhere, people walking or running on treadmills, people using ellipticals, people pedaling and spinning on bicycles, and swimmers doing laps. Widespread interest in cardio began in the 1970s when reports began to cite the health benefits of exercise. Before then, you never saw anyone running in the streets, and there were not millions of people of all ages running marathons. Fitness centers were extremely rare, and where they existed, the emphasis was almost exclusively on weightlifting.

Do you have to become a marathoner and train to run 26.2 miles to take advantage of cardiovascular conditioning? No, there are many ways to fulfill your weekly quota of cardio exercise that are far less strenuous and far less time-consuming. You may choose to walk or jog at a good pace outside or on a treadmill, use an elliptical machine or skiing simulator, use an indoor or outdoor bicycle, or swim laps. Just be sure it is a rhythmic exercise that increases your heartbeat, and that you can sustain it for at least 15 or 20 minutes (ideally, though, 30 minutes or more).

Below, we will answer your questions about the benefits of cardio conditioning, and you can learn how to start incorporating an agreeable form of cardio into your regular exercise routine.

1. **What are the health benefits of cardio exercise?**

    The news about the disease preventative potential of cardiovascular exercise is everywhere. You can't miss the countless articles, health reports, and TV programs emphasizing the importance of getting up and getting moving by raising your pulse and breathing deeply for at least 20 minutes.

A continuing stream of new studies and clinical trials cite the role of cardiovascular exercise in helping to prevent heart disease, including slowing the buildup of arterial plaque to reduce the risk of heart attacks and lowering high blood pressure to help prevent strokes. Cardio conditioning is also credited with preventing type 2 diabetes by lowering blood sugar and improving insulin resistance. Further, it may possibly prevent respiratory and digestive disorders and even reduce the risk of some forms of cancer. Aerobics are believed to strengthen the immune system, too.

The onset and progression of cognitive disorders, like dementia and Alzheimer's, are believed to be slowed by sustaining cardiovascular exercise. Even a long-term practice of walking a certain distance at a brisk pace at least three or four times per week is a health benefit.

2. **Does cardio help with weight control?**

One-third of Americans are classified as overweight, and another one-third are obese. These classifications are based on body mass index levels, which take height, weight, and gender into consideration. But, with cardio conditioning, you can get your weight down to a healthier level, since the calories burned during a cardio routine add up.

A robust 30- to 45-minute cardio workout can burn 400 to 500 calories, which helps chip away at excess pounds and keeps them off. Don't worry about burning off protein; your body uses carbohydrates (in the form of glycogen) for energy, and if that runs short (like during a long run), it burns fat.

3. **Does cardio provide psychological benefits?**

Cardio workouts can induce the release of beta-endorphins, the hormone that brings on the famous "runner's high." It's a medically verified effect and can relieve tension and stress, getting rid of both anxiety and depression.

You may now be wondering if a hard calisthenics workout can bring on the release of beta-endorphins. Very possibly, especially if the workout is conducted at a brisk pace. But the sustained intensity of a cardio workout seems to be more effective and consistent in creating the runner's high. When calisthenics and cardio are combined during the same workout period, the psychological and physical benefits are cumulative.

Aerobics are also credited with improving your mood by enlarging the hippocampus, the part of the brain that regulates emotion. It also can help you get a good night's sleep. Aerobics combined with calisthenics can improve brain plasticity to improve learning ability and memory as well.

4. Will cardiovascular conditioning help you to live longer?

Since it is credited with preventing or slowing the onset of so many life-threatening diseases and conditions, it is possible that cardio conditioning can help you live longer. But, to be objective, there are no guarantees in life, especially when our genetic profiles have so much influence. The responsible attitude is to do your best to improve the odds and give your body the fighting chance to survive and prosper for as long and as well as possible. Many marathoners believe that keeping in good cardiovascular condition may not necessarily put more years into your life, but it will definitely put more life into your years.

5. Do you need a doctor's approval?

It's recommended by medical and fitness professionals that you consult with your doctor before beginning any strenuous activity, especially if you have not had a thorough physical examination within the past year.

It's a good idea to get the heart and circulatory system checked out, and chances are very good that you will be encouraged to begin both calisthenic and cardio training with the advice to start gradually at first, take it easy, and work up to greater intensity over time.

Beware of your body's warnings during cardio workouts, especially pain in your chest, shoulder, or left arm, which could be a signal, like angina, that the blood flow to your heart is being impeded or blocked. Stop exercising if that happens and call your doctor.

6. **How much cardio exercise do you need?**

The current consensus is that at least three days per week of brisk walking or jogging, biking, elliptical, or swimming are sufficient, but four or more days is preferable.

If the pace is moderate, a total of 150 minutes per week is a good base level. If the pace is brisk with deeper breathing and getting the pulse rate up, 75 to 100 minutes per week is a good base. But some fitness enthusiasts push up to 300 minutes per week.

When you are in good condition, the quality of the cardio workout can be enhanced by doing intervals, which are bursts of speed and/or increased incline. The interval should last for 20 to 40 seconds, during which time you are really working hard. After the interval, you slow back down and take two minutes of rest before the next interval. A total of six to eight intervals during the workout will add considerable conditioning benefits.

Since you have now chosen your plan and put together your initial strategy for sticking with that plan, we are ready to advance and discuss progression and how to increase the tension and difficulty of your bodyweight calisthenics exercises.

Chapter 7:

Progression

The overall objective of your calisthenics workout plan is to get you started easily and immediately and then to start the transition to more intensive levels. First, you will work through three basic levels, then up to two intermediate levels, and, finally, you'll step up and transition to the first advanced level.

When to progress to a higher level of intensity or a more complex form of an exercise movement depends on you. Factors to consider are your perception of your level of expertise, the ability to perform each exercise correctly (in good form), the ability to complete the recommended number of reps and sets, and the will to follow the recommended timing for each cycle of the movements and rest duration between sets.

You should follow your own sense of progress, but here is a suggested 18-week timeline that covers your first six 21-day cycles. This timeline is based on typical progress and assumes a complete commitment to performing all nine of the exercises correctly and completely and adhering to their workouts schedule.

1st 21 Days	2nd 21 Days	3rd 21 Days

Week 1	Week 2	Week 3	Week 4	Week 5	Week 6	Week 7	Week 8	Week 9
Basic 1	Basic 1	Basic 1 or 2	Basic 2	Basic 2	Basic 2 or 3	Basic 3	Basic 3	Basic 3
4th 21 Days			5th 21 Days			6th 21 Days		
Week 10	Week 11	Week 12	Week 13	Week 14	Week 15	Week 16	Week 17	Week 18
Inter 1	Inter 1	Inter 1	Inter 2	Inter 2	Inter 2	Advance 1	Advance 1	Advance 1

Mastering the Basic Levels

Basic Level 1

This is where you will begin: Basic Level 1 on Day 1 of Week 1. This is the 21-day plan from the previous chapter that follows the one-day-on/two-days-off pattern where you perform all nine exercises during one session. This plan provides seven workout days and 14 rest/recovery days during each 21-day cycle. Consider this the foundation from which you will advance in the coming weeks and months.

Begins Week 1

Day 1

Movement	Muscle Groups	Reps	Sets	Cycle Time *	Between Sets	21 Day Schedule
Pull-Ups	Upper Body	6	3	3-4 seconds	90 seconds	1 - 4 - 7 - 10 - 13 - 16 - 19
Leg Raises	Core Lower Body	6	3	5 seconds	90 seconds	1 - 4 - 7 - 10 - 13 - 16 - 19
Superman	Core, Upper Lower Body	6	3	3 seconds	60 seconds	1 - 4 - 7 - 10 - 13 - 16 - 19
Dips	Upper Body	6	3	4 seco	90 second	1 - 4 - 7 -

				nds	s	10 - 13 - 16 - 19
Squats	Lower Body	6	3	4 seconds	60 seconds	1 - 4 - 7 - 10 - 13 - 16 - 19
Push-Ups	Upper Body Core	8	3	4 seconds	90 seconds	1 - 4 - 7 - 10 - 13 - 16 - 19
Calf Raises	Lower Body	14	3	8 seconds	30 seconds	1 - 4 - 7 - 10 - 13 - 16 - 19
Side Planks	Upper Body Core	1 each side	3	30 seconds	90 seconds	1 - 4 - 7 - 10 - 13 - 16 - 19
Chin-Ups	Upper Body	6	3	3-4 seconds	90 seconds	1 - 4 - 7 - 10 - 13 - 16 - 19

Basic Level 2

After about two weeks of following Basic Level 1, you should be ready to work a little harder and move onto Basic Level 2. The number of reps increases for most exercises during this level, which begins in either week 3 or week 4, depending on individual progress. Only the side plank remains the same at one rep per side, but the cycle timing is extended. There are no changes in sets or duration of rest time between sets for any of the exercises.

Begins Week 3 or 4

Day 22 or 29

Movement	Muscle Groups	Reps	Sets	Cycle Time *	Between Sets	21 Day Schedule
Pull-Ups	Upper Body	8	3	3-4 seconds	90 seconds	1 - 4 - 7 - 10 - 13 - 16 - 19
Leg Raises	Core Lower Body	10	3	5 seconds	90 seconds	1 - 4 - 7 - 10 - 13 - 16 - 19

Superman	Core, Upper Lower Body	8	3	3 seconds	60 seconds	1 - 4 - 7 - 10 - 13 - 16 - 19
Dips	Upper Body	8	3	4 seconds	90 seconds	1 - 4 - 7 - 10 - 13 - 16 - 19
Squats	Lower Body	10	3	4 seconds	60 seconds	1 - 4 - 7 - 10 - 13 - 16 - 19
Push-Ups	Upper Body Core	10	3	4 seconds	90 seconds	1 - 4 - 7 - 10 - 13 - 16 - 19
Calf Raises	Lower Body	18	3	8 seconds	30 seconds	1 - 4 - 7 - 10 - 13 - 16 - 19
Side Planks	Upper Body Core	1 each	3	40 seco	90 second	1 - 4 - 7 -

		side		nds	s	10 - 13 - 16 - 19
Chin-Ups	Upper Body	8	3	3-4 seconds	90 seconds	1 - 4 - 7 - 10 - 13 - 16 - 19

Basic Level 3

Basic Level 3 can begin in either week 6 or week 7, depending on individual progress. The number of reps does not change for any of the exercises, but the cycle time is extended for each exercise. By extending the time it takes to go up and down or down and up each time, the exercise will definitely start to feel harder. There are no changes in sets or rest between sets.

Begins Week 6 or 7

Day 43 or 50

Movement	Muscle Groups	Reps	Sets	Cycle Time *	Between Sets	21 Day Schedule
Pull-Ups	Upper Body	8	3	6-8	90	1 - 4 - 7 -

				seconds	seconds	10 - 13 - 16 - 19
Leg Raises	Core Lower Body	10	3	8 seconds	90 seconds	1 - 4 - 7 - 10 - 13 - 16 - 19
Superman	Core, Upper Lower Body	8	3	6 seconds	60 seconds	1 - 4 - 7 - 10 - 13 - 16 - 19
Dips	Upper Body	8	3	8 seconds	90 seconds	1 - 4 - 7 - 10 - 13 - 16 - 19
Squats	Lower Body	10	3	10 seconds	60 seconds	1 - 4 - 7 - 10 - 13 - 16 - 19
Push-Ups	Upper Body Core	10	3	8 seconds	90 seconds	1 - 4 - 7 - 10 - 13 - 16 - 19

Calf Raises	Lower Body	18	3	12-14 seconds	30 seconds	1 - 4 - 7 - 10 - 13 - 16 - 19
Side Planks	Upper Body Core	1 each side	3	50 seconds	90 seconds	1 - 4 - 7 - 10 - 13 - 16 - 19
Chin-Ups	Upper Body	8	3	6-8 seconds	90 seconds	1 - 4 - 7 - 10 - 13 - 16 - 19

Transitioning to Intermediate Level 1

By now, you should have mastered Basic Level 3 and are ready for the transition to Intermediate Level 1, which begins in week 10. The number of reps increases for most exercises here and the rest time between sets is reduced. Side planks remain at one rep per side, but the cycle timing is extended. There are no changes in the cycle time or number of sets.

Begins Week 10

Day 71

Movement	Muscle Groups	Reps	Sets	Cycle Time *	Between Sets	21 Day Schedule
Pull-Ups	Upper Body	12-14	3	6-8 seconds	60 seconds	1 - 4 - 7 - 10 - 13 - 16 - 19
Leg Raises	Core, Lower Body	18-24	3	8 seconds	60 seconds	1 - 4 - 7 - 10 - 13 - 16 - 19
Superman	Core, Upper Lower Body	12-14	3	6 seconds	50 seconds	1 - 4 - 7 - 10 - 13 - 16 - 19
Dips	Upper Body	14-16	3	8 seconds	60 seconds	1 - 4 - 7 - 10 - 13 - 16 - 19
Squats	Lower	16-	3	10	50	1 - 4 - 7

	Body	22		seconds	seconds	- 10 - 13 - 16 - 19
Push-Ups	Upper Body Core	20-26	3	8 seconds	60 seconds	1 - 4 - 7 - 10 - 13 - 16 - 19
Calf Raises	Lower Body	24-30	3	12-14 seconds	20 seconds	1 - 4 - 7 - 10 - 13 - 16 - 19
Side Planks	Upper Body Core	1 each side	3	60 seconds	60 seconds	1 - 4 - 7 - 10 - 13 - 16 - 19
Chin-Ups	Upper Body	12-16	3	6-8 seconds	60 seconds	1 - 4 - 7 - 10 - 13 - 16 - 19

Intermediate Level 2

Intermediate Level 2 begins in week 13. The number of reps does not change for any of the exercises but the cycle time is extended for some exercise. There are no changes in sets or rest between sets. You should find the longer cycle times having a noticeable effect in making the exercises harder.

Begins Week 13

Day 92

Movement	Muscle Groups	Reps	Sets	Cycle Time *	Between Sets	21 Day Schedule
Pull-Ups	Upper Body	10-12	3	6-8 seconds	60 seconds	1 - 4 - 7 - 10 - 13 - 16 - 19
Leg Raises	Core, Lower Body	14-20	3	10 seconds	60 seconds	1 - 4 - 7 - 10 - 13 - 16 - 19
Superman	Core, Upper, Lower Body	10-12	3	10 seconds	50 seconds	1 - 4 - 7 - 10 - 13 - 16 -

						19
Dips	Upper Body	10-12	3	10 seconds	60 seconds	1 - 4 - 7 - 10 - 13 - 16 - 19
Squats	Lower Body	12-16	3	10 seconds	50 seconds	1 - 4 - 7 - 10 - 13 - 16 - 19
Push-Ups	Upper Body Core	14-18	3	10 seconds	60 seconds	1 - 4 - 7 - 10 - 13 - 16 - 19
Calf Raises	Lower Body	20-24	3	16 seconds	20 seconds	1 - 4 - 7 - 10 - 13 - 16 - 19
Side Planks	Upper Body Core	1 each side	3	60 seconds	60 seconds	1 - 4 - 7 - 10 - 13 - 16 - 19
Chin-	Upper	10-	3	6-8	60	1 - 4 - 7

Ups	Body	12		seconds	seconds	- 10 - 13 - 16 - 19

Transitioning to Advanced Level 1

If your workouts have been following the schedule and you have progressed through the Basic and Intermediate Levels, you should be ready to begin Advanced Level 1. If you think you are not yet up to it and need more time at one of the Intermediate Levels, relax and take the time to repeat a cycle. There's no rush, and you should progress at your own speed. Remember, we're all different and no two people will build muscles and strength at the same rate. Advanced Level 1 begins in week 16. The number of reps and the cycle times do not change for any of the exercises, but the number of sets increases from three to four for each exercise. There are no changes in the rest time between sets.

Begins Week 16

Day 113

Movement	Muscle Groups	Reps	Sets	Cycle Time	Between Sets	21 Day Schedule

				e *		
Pull-Ups	Upper Body	10-12	4	6-8 seconds	60 seconds	1 - 4 - 7 - 10 - 13 - 16 - 19
Leg Raises	Core Lower Body	14-20	4	10 seconds	60 seconds	1 - 4 - 7 - 10 - 13 - 16 - 19
Superman	Core, Upper Lower Body	10-12	4	10 seconds	50 seconds	1 - 4 - 7 - 10 - 13 - 16 - 19
Dips	Upper Body	10-12	4	10 seconds	60 seconds	1 - 4 - 7 - 10 - 13 - 16 - 19
Squats	Lower Body	12-16	4	10 seconds	50 seconds	1 - 4 - 7 - 10 - 13 - 16 - 19
Push-	Upper	14-	4	10	60	1 - 4 - 7

Ups	Body Core	18		seconds	seconds	- 10 - 13 - 16 - 19
Calf Raises	Lower Body	20-24	4	16 seconds	20 seconds	1 - 4 - 7 - 10 - 13 - 16 - 19
Side Planks	Upper Bod, Core	1 each side	4	60 seconds	60 seconds	1 - 4 - 7 - 10 - 13 - 16 - 19
Chin-Ups	Upper Body	10-12	4	6-8 seconds	60 seconds	1 - 4 - 7 - 10 - 13 - 16 - 19

Transitioning to Advanced Level 2 and More Advanced Calisthenics

After completing the Basic Level, Intermediate Level, and Advanced Level 2 18-week schedule, you may feel you are ready to integrate compound versions of the current nine exercises into your routine and/or take on more difficult versions of the exercises. Advanced Level 2 and beyond is where you begin training for maximum results by challenging your body and mind.

Pull-Ups and Chin-Ups with Leg Raises

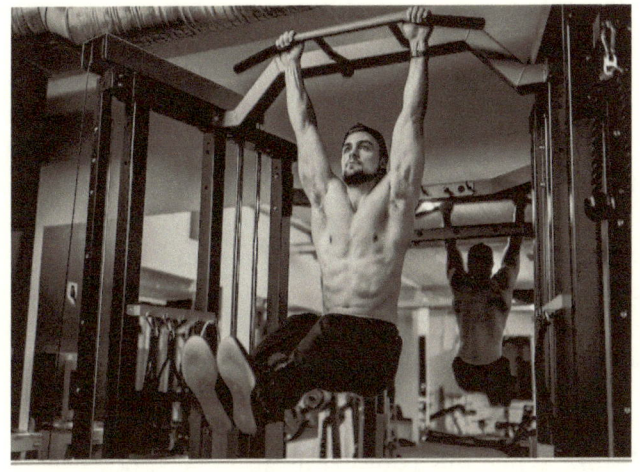

Fig. 11

Where: Like a regular pull-up or chin-up, for this exercise, you will need a horizontal bar that is at the height of your extended arms.

How: This is a compound exercise, which employs two separate movements to increase the work done within a given time and to engage and challenge multiple muscle groups. If doing pull-ups, grasp the bar with both hands with palms forward and arms shoulder width apart. If doing chin-ups, reverse the grip so your palms face backward. As you pull slowly upward, raise your legs and fully extend them until they are parallel to the ground if possible (or lift as far as you can). When you reach the bar with your head, pause and slowly lower back down while also slowly lowering your legs to the vertical (downward position). Repeat the pull-up or chin and leg raise cycle as many times as you can while doing the exercise correctly and in good form.

The leg raises can be made *easier* by pulling your knees up to your chest (as shown in the image above), instead of extending the legs fully outward. It can be made *harder* by maintaining the legs in the fully raised position (parallel to the ground) as you raise and lower for the required number of cycles.

Link to the video demo: https://www.youtube.com/watch?v=QyVq5oUBpss

Result: While this is primarily an upper-body exercise, the leg raises engage the core, the abdominal, the back muscle groups, the hip flexors, and the quadriceps.

Horizontal Rows

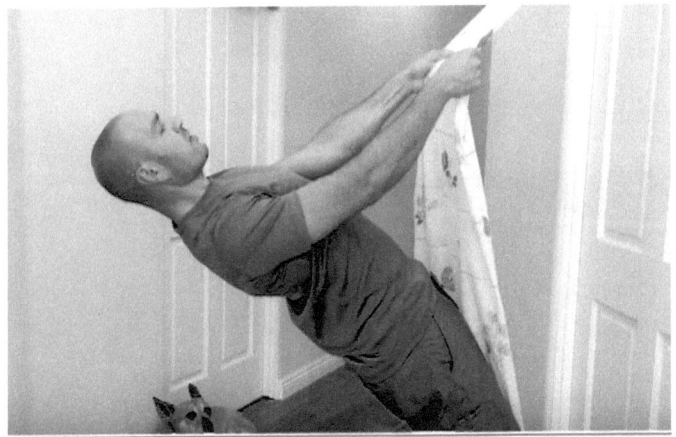

Fig. 12

Where: Horizontal rows can be performed at home, using ordinary furniture, using a lowered chinning bar, or simply using a sheet in a doorway (as seen above).

How: One version is to slide under a table and, while facing upward, reach up to the edge of the table and pull upward. Alternatively, you can use a sheet that is held firmly in place in a doorway, as shown in the video demo. You hold onto the sheet while leaning backward, and with arms held apart, lower yourself and raise back up. Do as many cycles of this exercise as you can until fatigued, rest 60 seconds, and perform two more sets.

Link to the video demo:
https://www.youtube.com/watch?v=rloXYB8M3vU

Result: Trainers encourage horizontal rows to improve posture and to strengthen the arms, shoulders, and core for pull-ups and chin-ups.

Reverse Grip Horizontal Row

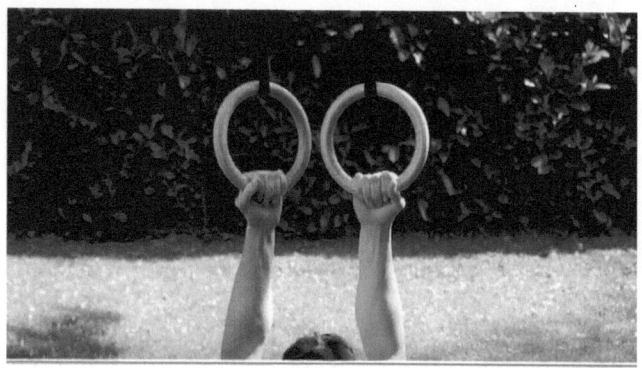

Fig. 13

Where: At home or in a fitness center where you can hold onto a bar or a set of rings, as you can see in the demo video.

How: There are variations of the grip, including forward (as seen above) or backward. Your hands can also be in both forward and back positions. You will see these reverse and regular grip examples in the demo. You perform the horizontal row by holding onto the ring or bar, leaning back, and pulling yourself upright again.

Link to the video demo:
https://www.youtube.com/watch?v=PGcTxvw6-lo

Results: Reverse and regular horizontal rows build the upper back muscles, especially the rhomboids, lats, traps, rear delts, and the upper arms (notably, the biceps).

Diamond Push-Up

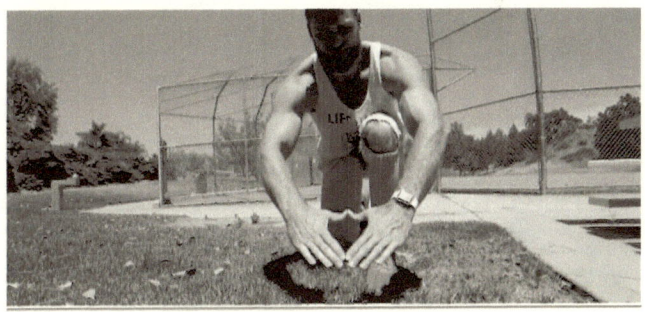

Fig. 14

Where: As with regular push-ups, this exercise may be performed indoors or outdoors on a flat, even surface.

How: Assume a normal push-up position, facing downward with your body fully extended and your arms holding you up, but instead of placing your hands under your shoulders, move your hands together so that they form a diamond shape with thumbs and index fingers touching (see above). Shift your weight forward so your hands are beneath your sternum.

Link to the video demo:
https://www.youtube.com/watch?v=ZR5U3sb-KeE

Results: With your hands together and your arms close to your body, the diamond push-up works the triceps, the delts, and other chest muscles.

Handstand Push-Up

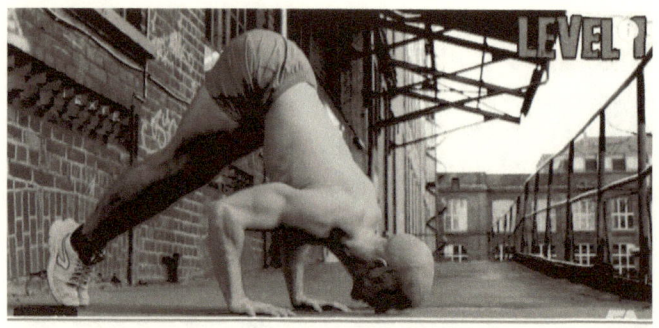

Fig. 15

Where: The handstand push-up may be performed indoors or out on a flat service or by gripping two parallel bars. It may be advisable to do this exercise close to a wall, which can assist with balance when you are first trying the movement.

How: This is a difficult and challenging exercise, but it can be rewarding if you work through it and progress gradually in stages. As shown in the image and as you will see in the demo video, you may begin with level 1 with your body bent forward and your feet still on the ground. Position yourself so your chest and abdominals will be facing the wall. As your routine progresses through subsequent stages, you will be placing your feet on the wall for support and balance and working your way up to be increasingly vertical. Eventually, your goal will be to push up and lower down in a balanced, vertical position, without touching the wall.

Link to the video demo:
https://www.youtube.com/watch?v=h0HjqYRlXYg

Results: This is one of the most effective exercises to build your triceps, upper arms, and shoulders. Muscle groups throughout the core are engaged, especially the back.

One-Arm Push-Up/Archer Push-Up

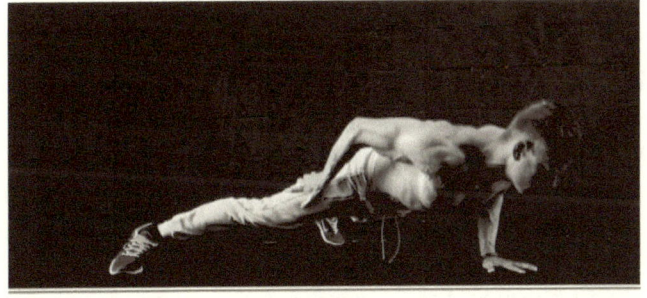

Fig. 16

Where: Any floor or flat surface will be satisfactory.

How: Assume the basic starting push-up position but then place your hands a bit closer together to help maintain your balance. Lift one arm and rest in on the hips. Using only the remaining arm, lower yourself and keep your body from sagging or twisting. Control the movements with your arms, shoulders, core, and legs. Do not let your back arch or sway. Don't turn your body or dip your shoulder downward during the descent movement. Keep your body horizontal.

The archer push-up is a variation that uses both arms but keeps most of the tension on one arm. As you will see in the demo, one arm remains vertical, as in the one arm movement, but the other arm is extended to the side with the hand on the floor. The extended arm takes some of the pressure off the vertical arm. This is one way to ease gradually into the full one-arm pull-up.

Link to the video demo: https://www.youtube.com/watch?v=KIEAbfk4cQU

Results: When you have reached the stage where you can do many repetitions of the basic push-up, the one-arm push-up will enable you to have a hard, challenging workout. Among other benefits, performing push-ups unilaterally will reveal if one side is weaker than the other and needs compensatory training. You will achieve the benefits of regular, two-arm push-ups with far fewer repetitions. Shoulders, arms, and all parts of the core will benefit.

Straight Bar Dip and Parallel Bars Dip

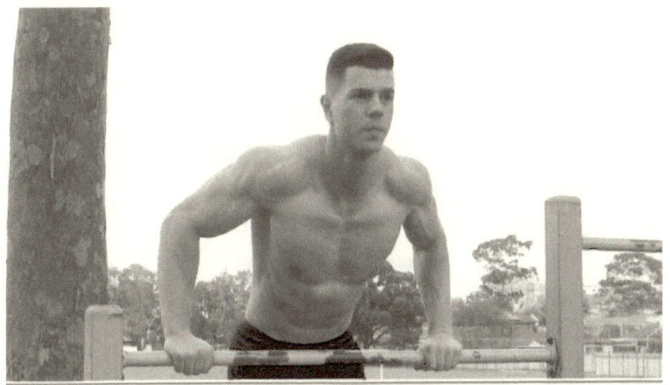

Fig. 17

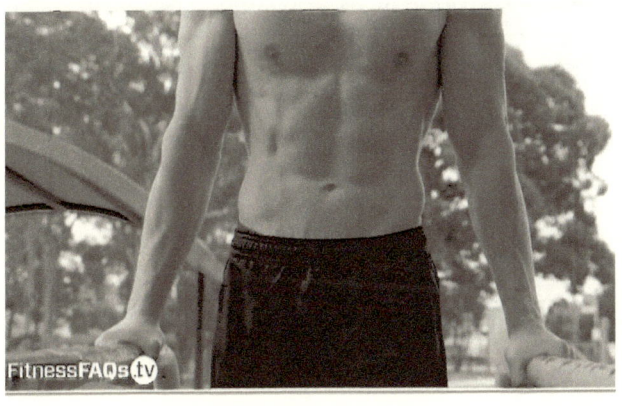

Fig. 18

Where: To perform dips on a bar, a single (straight) bar or double (parallel) bars are needed.

How: The dips are performed by placing hands on the straight bar or by standing between the parallel bars and placing one hand on each bar. Push the weight of your body up until the arms are straight, dip down by bending the arms, pause, and then push back up to complete one cycle. Parallel bar dips are believed to work the muscles, including the triceps, more correctly with a more upright position and a fuller lowering, and they are safer and less likely to lead to injury. Perform eight reps at a slow pace or an amount you can handle without excessive effort or strain.

Link to the video demo:
https://www.youtube.com/watch?v=2IUoEAzjZqY

Benefits: Both straight bar dips and parallel bar dips are beneficial to the arms, the shoulders, and the chest, but compared to parallel bar dips, straight bar dips give you more internal core rotation and put more tension on the pectoral (chest) muscles.

Tucked Planche Progressions

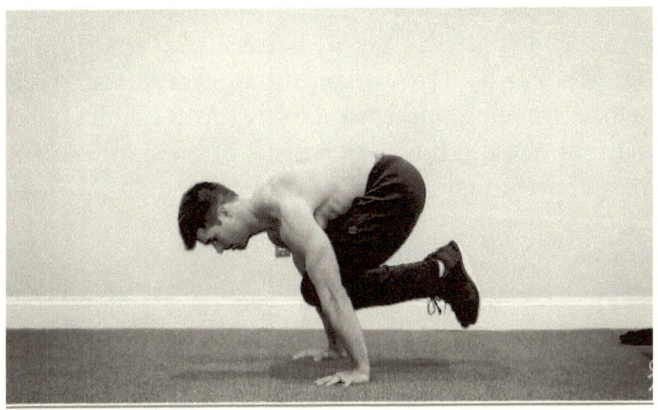

Fig. 19

Where: Like push-ups and other floor-based exercises, the tucked planche may be performed on any flat surface.

How: The tucked planche is often considered difficult, but with the right set-up technique, it can be mastered. It is a great calisthenic exercise and worth learning as part of your advanced levels. Warm-up by stretching the hamstring muscles by bending over and touching the toes or extending one leg and bending toward your knee. Lower yourself to your stomach and rise up on your arms to stretch the core (the yoga cobra pose). Then, sit back on your heels, fold forward, and stretch your arms forward (child's pose) to stretch the lower back. Stand up and then crouch down, knees far apart, lean forward, and place your hands on the floor. Place your elbows inside your knees and roll gently forward until your feet are off the floor and your entire weight is being held up by your arms and shoulders. It will take some practice to achieve the balance you need to hold the position and to make the progressions, which include swinging one knee into the center and to drop one foot one the floor. All aspects of these movements are well presented in the demo video.

Link to the video demo:
https://www.youtube.com/watch?v=iT1q1Ff02mk

Results: The tucked planche is highly beneficial to the core and the shoulders. It also develops the triceps, the chest, and the muscles of the serratus anterior, helping to prevent poor posture.

Lateral Lunge

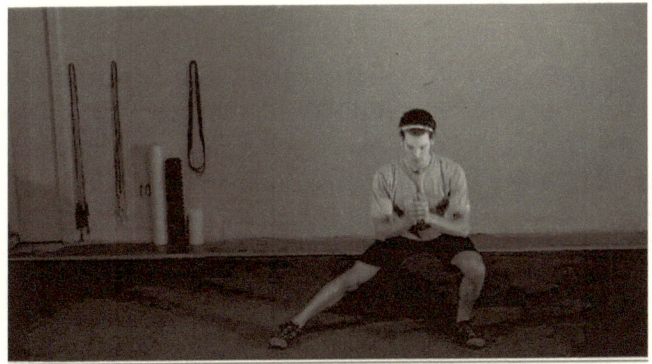

Fig. 20

Where: Lateral lunges may be performed on a level surface indoors or outside, ensuring there is ample space for you to take long steps sideways.

How: Stand upright with your feet spaced about 18 inches apart. With your left leg, step to the left side, about three feet, and squat down on the right leg. Keep your weight back and toward the glutes. Pause for a second and then push back up to the standing position. Repeat the movement on the left side. Maintain your balance by keeping your body upright throughout the exercise. Perform eight reps to begin and increase to 12 reps as you progress. Perform two or three sets with a 60-second rest interval.

Link to the video demo:
https://www.youtube.com/watch?v=gwWv7aPcD88

Results: The lateral lunge is a simple but effective movement to strengthen the quadriceps, the glutes, and the hip flexors.

With your plan in full movement, you may run into some concerns. So, the following chapter will address some troubleshooting issues and FAQs that may arise as you move through your bodyweight calisthenics program.

Chapter 8:

Troubleshooting

In any instructional book, questions may arise that are not addressed in the explanations and instructions, so the objective of this chapter is to anticipate your possible questions and problems and provide answers and solutions. Before getting started, let's remind ourselves of some fundamentals that may head off your concerns.

First, Do No Harm

While bodyweight calisthenics exercises are considered safer and less likely to cause injury compared to weightlifting, do not underestimate the risks of overuse injuries, pulls, tears, and strains. Listen to your body, and don't overdo it. If you are trying to do 12 pushups and are having trouble getting past number eight and your shoulders are crying out, take it easy and don't force yourself to do them in pain. Even if you had done 12 reps a few days ago or during a previous set, this time you may have run out of steam. And that's okay. A few days of rest may be all you need to get back to 12 reps.

Look at it this way: If you work up to a point that it starts to really hurt or you are having difficulty completing the movements in good form, it means your muscles have been pushed far enough for that moment, so back off and let them begin to rest and recover. Pain can also signal a small injury that you might make worse if you continue to challenge the muscles or joints.

It is very important not to push beyond your physical limits, which you can do by performing too many reps, exercising in bad form, not resting between sets, not allowing the full two days to recover between workouts, or assuming a position that puts an unbearable strain on a joint, a ligament, or muscle group.

You Are Unique

No two people have the same DNA (except identical twins), and that means no two people have the same skills, strengths, competencies, and endurance. Everyone has different cognitive and mental capacities as well. So, we should not expect to do exactly what others can do. We based the Basic, Intermediate, and Advanced levels for reps, sets, cycle speeds, and rest time between sets on averages and the experience of countless coaches, trainers, and sports medicine professionals. But they are only estimates meant to guide you and are not hard and fast criteria you must meet.

How you build muscles with bulk and with definition will be unique to your physiology. You should respect your body's particular qualities. Be assured that if you work at this program, you will build muscles, grow stronger, and be more physically fit.

Give Your Muscles Time to Build

The process of working your muscles hard so that cells and fibers are damaged and need to rebuild is a gradual process. While you may feel "pumped up" and muscular immediately after a hard workout, that's the temporary pooling of blood and other fluids; it will subside after a few hours. The real growth of muscle tissue takes place slowly and microscopically, so don't expect your muscles to grow to a bulging size within days. But over weeks and months, the growth of your upper body, core, and lower body muscles will become apparent. Give it time.

Bodyweight Calisthenics Q&As

With that preamble behind us, here are answers to specific questions you may have.

Q: Are calisthenics a real fitness workout?

A: Calisthenics comprise a distinct and recognized form of physical training that is meant to build muscles and strength by using one's own bodyweight instead of weights, machines, and other forms of equipment (other than a bar for pull-ups, chin-ups, and rows). Calisthenics can build muscle by adding bulk, strength, and definition. But unlike some other forms of exercise, it also contributes to flexibility and functionality by not making you muscle bound, inflexible and/or tight.

Calisthenics can be easily learned, and the workouts can be performed anywhere. Do not let the simplicity and ease of access to calisthenics cause you to underestimate its potential to create a great physique or underestimate the value of using your own bodyweight. Even if you weigh just 90 pounds, you'll be impressed when your workout has you lifting some or all of that 90 pounds!

Q: Do I need special preparation to get started with bodyweight calisthenics?

A: If you are in reasonably good health, you should be able to begin training immediately—today—if you want. The Basic Level plans intentionally start you off with a low level of reps and gradually increases reps and shortens rest times so that you will advance at a reasonable pace.

If you are unsure if your health is up to the challenge, it's advisable to check with your doctor; a physical exam may be appropriate. This is especially important if you are also beginning cardiovascular exercise.

Q: Can calisthenics really build muscles?

A: When we're referring to bodyweight calisthenics, as presented in this book, the answer is an unequivocal "yes." Some people associate calisthenics with stretching, jumping jacks, skipping rope, and/or cardio training. But bodyweight calisthenics are a highly effective, cost-free, and safe way to build muscles for added bulk and definition. Bodyweight resistance creates the process we call hypertrophy: physical tension and metabolic stress that damages muscle fibers and cells, leading to more rebuilt muscle tissue than was lost and creating muscle growth.

Q: Is bodyweight calisthenics training better than weight training?

A: No, it is just different. But weight training is not better than calisthenics, either. Both weight lifting and bodyweight calisthenics work to achieve the same primary goals of building muscle and strength. Lifting weights and using resistance equipment are very effective at creating hypertrophy and may bulk you up a little faster. But that is offset by calisthenics being less likely to cause injury and not needing access to a gym or fitness center.

Some advanced calisthenics enthusiasts will bring some weights and resistance machines into their routines. For example, doing squats while holding a pair of dumbbells or a barbell. We recommend you focus exclusively on calisthenics initially, and if you continue to increase reps, slow cycle times, and shorten rest between sets, you will continue to challenge your muscles and grow muscle bulk and strength. You can also graduate to the more advanced calisthenics exercises that are shown in chapter 7.

Q: *How often should I conduct my workouts?*

A: As we discussed in chapters 6 and 7, a top priority is for you to allow adequate time for recovery between workouts, and this was determined to be at least two rest days between workouts. The 21-day plans offer two exercise scheduling options: Performing all nine calisthenics exercises in one session ("nine-in-one") or doing some calisthenics on one day and the remaining group of exercises the next day ("nine-in-two"). In either case, the muscles that are worked are not engaged and challenged again until they have had two days of rest.

For example, with the nine-in-one schedule, if your workout is on Monday, you would rest and do no bodyweight calisthenics on Tuesday or Wednesday and return to all nine exercises on Thursday. If you want to put three days between calisthenics exercises, that's okay. But do not put too much separation between sessions or you will start to lose some strength and it will be more difficult to get back to the exercise. So to sum it up: Each muscle group should be exercised two or three times a week.

Q: Can I do bodyweight calisthenics and cardiovascular workouts on the same day?

A: Yes, it is commonly done, especially when both are completed in the same facility like a fitness center or gym. Many people find it convenient and satisfying to "get it all done" in the same extended session. The satisfaction is also due to the increased flow of beta-endorphins. The combination of cardio and resistance exercises is cumulative, or synergistic, meaning the end result is equal to or greater than the sum of the parts.

Most people who are into both forms of exercise prefer to do the cardio workout first, immediately followed by calisthenics. Why? Cardio warms up the entire body by increasing circulation to virtually every cell and muscle in the body, while calisthenics increases circulation to the muscle group being worked. Following cardio with calisthenics ensures that all the muscle groups are already warmed up, making it easier to get going. Conversely, if you exercised your lower body first, you might find it harder to push forward with cardio exercises that are working the quadriceps, the hamstrings, the calves, and the hip flexors.

Q: Should I do my workout if I am injured or in pain?

A: Short answer: no. As we said at the beginning of this chapter, "First, do no harm," (which is borrowed from the Hippocratic oath that doctors recite upon receiving their license to practice). But it is worth repeating that there is no advantage to pushing yourself when in real pain, which is a warning that you are injured or soon to be injured. If you feel pain in a muscle or joint, try to work through it slowly, testing it to determine if it's something that you can manage, something that needs rest, or something serious that a healthcare professional should examine.

All the same, it's important to recognize minor discomforts (soreness, stiffness, or the muscle burn of working out) and learn how to work through them. It's natural to have a little soreness left over from the last workout. One of the side effects of post-workout recovery is the buildup of lactate, or lactic acid, in the muscle cells. This is a natural byproduct of muscle work, and until it dissipates, it can cause some stiffness and soreness. It's not harmful, and you just may need to go a little easier when it bothers you. Be sure to allow enough recovery time between workouts, and there is certainly no harm in delaying the workout for another day.

Q: Will calisthenics help me lose weight?

A: You can expect to lose weight if the amount of calories you burn is greater than the amount of calories you consume. There is no shortcut or exception to this fundamental rule of science. Your metabolism, which is the rate your body uses energy, is unique to you, which means no two people use up calories at the same rate. So, two people on the identical diet and on the identical workout schedule may vary in their weight gains or losses.

Generally, a good calisthenics workout will burn 200 to 400 calories. If the rest of your physical activities remain the same and you include calisthenics workouts in your routine, then, over a couple of weeks, that can add up to as much as a pound of weight loss. Over a year, it can mean some serious slimming.

But there are some additional factors to consider. More muscle bulk can add more pounds, since muscle is denser than the fat it is replacing. Also, after working out, whether it's with calisthenics or cardio, your metabolism slows down, especially when resting, so the net calorie loss for the day may be less than you think. Reducing the calories in your diet in combination with exercise is the single most effective way to lose weight. Refer to chapter 2's coverage of nutrition and the Mediterranean diet to review the best sources for calories.

Q: What if I can't do all of the reps in the Basic or Intermediate 21-Day Plans?

A: As explained, the plans are recommendations based on averages and extensive experience, but you should follow your own abilities and do the number of reps for each exercise that challenges you, but you should know when to stop. Generally, between eight to 12 reps should be the ideal amount with the last two reps feeling really tough but doable without wrecking your form. Bad form includes kicking your way toward the chin-up bar or doing your push-ups without lowering all the way down. Use the "last two" being tough as your guide to when to stop. If you are straining to get rep number eight completed in good form and without doing the movement sloppily, that should be your stopping point.

Be aware of the rest time you are taking between sets as well. If your place in the plan has you resting for 60 seconds, you may need to raise it back to the original 90 seconds or even to two minutes, if it will enable you to complete more reps.

Q: What if the number of reps in the plans are not enough? Can I do more?

A: Again, as mentioned in the previous answer, the 21-day plans are recommendations, not firm rules, and you should recognize your own abilities. When the number of reps is not enough to cause you to reach the "last two" being tough, you have three options to consider:

1. **Do more reps.** Just be sure you are performing all reps correctly with full ups and downs, with a straight back, and with good form and posture. Also, be sure that you are not taking shortcuts.
2. **Shorten the rest time between sets.** For example, lower the 60 seconds to 30 seconds of rest between sets. You should find the reps

getting harder to do when your rest time between sets is shorter.
3. **Slow the cycle rate of each rep so that each movement takes longer.** For example, taking 12 seconds to perform one push-up cycle or slowing down and taking 10 seconds for one complete chin-up or pull-up.

Q: What if I am not seeing the results I am expecting?

A: First, refer to the sections at the start of this chapter entitled "You are Unique" and "Give Your Muscles Time to Build." These explain how you develop muscles at a unique pace and why you need to have patience before seeing the results you are hoping for.

But this is not to imply that you should lower your expectations for a good physique and greater strength. The series of 21-day plans will definitely get you there, even if it may take longer than you think. What is most important is that you follow the plans as best as you can, doing the hard work during each calisthenics session and allowing sufficient rest and recovery time between workouts. You also want to ensure that you have enough protein in your diet to fuel the rebuilding of muscle fibers.

If you push through the 21-day plans, do more reps, perform the reps more slowly, add sets, and shorten rest time between sets, you may shorten the time it takes to get bulkier, more cut-looking muscular results. The harder you work your muscles, the faster they will rebuild larger and stronger. Just pay attention to your physical limits to avoid injury, and be sure to maintain at least two days of recovery between workouts to let the repair and rebuilding process run its full cycle.

Things You Might Be Doing Wrong

There are some other factors that could be slowing you down in reaching your muscle and strength building goals. These include diet, sleep, stress, and both underwork and overwork.

1. **Protein**

    We've mentioned diet in the above section, but let's focus on protein. Are you getting enough? It can be difficult because meat is one of the best sources of protein, yet for cardiovascular health, we are encouraged to limit red meat consumption. But that refers to meat covered with and marbled through with saturated fats.

    Stick with lean, fat-free or low-fat servings of beef, turkey, chicken, and pork. Trim any visible fat before cooking. Fish is an even superior source of quality protein, plus other nutrients and antioxidants, so include fish in your diet at least twice a week.

However, there are other important protein sources apart from meat and fish. Choose vegetables, nuts, whole grains, and beans with high protein content. Also, include eggs and fat-free or low -at dairy in your diet. If you like yogurt, choose the Greek or Icelandic versions, which are very high in protein (18 to 19 grams of protein in a ¾ cup serving). If you remember from chapter 2, a normal adult needs about 50 grams of protein per day, but as a muscle-builder, you need at least 100 grams per day. Some serious calisthenics and weightlifting enthusiasts take in up to 150 grams of protein daily; although, that's a bit excessive for most of us. You need sufficient protein so that your body has enough available to do all the rebuilding your workouts make necessary.

2. **Sleep**

Are you getting enough sleep to enable your body to repair itself?

Everyone needs a good night's sleep. First, our brains need to process all of the day's impressions and inputs by letting our 100 billion neurons readjust their trillions of neural connections and flood the cells and neurons with the cleansing fluids and enzymes that remove potentially toxic wastes and plaques that can mess with cognitive abilities. We dream during sleep and need that time to further clear up and sort thoughts and memories.

Additionally, when we sleep, much of the repairing and rebuilding of our damaged muscles takes place. It's the ideal time since the muscles are inactive and the repair process has minimal interruptions. But if you do not get the requisite amount of sleep every night, the repairs will be interrupted or diminished, which will slow your bodybuilding progress.

This is worth thinking about: All that hard calisthenics exercise and the needed rebuilding is interrupted due to bad sleep habits. See chapter 3's discussion of sleep and remind yourself that eight hours every night is ideal. Take note of the steps that will help you fall asleep and stay asleep. Especially, plan to go to bed at the same time every night and wake at the same time every morning. And leave the digital devices out of the bedroom!

3. **Stress**

Are you experiencing continuing stress or anxiety in your life?

It happens to all of us. Stress is actually a normal reaction to danger or risk, and it's the central nervous system's self-protection mechanism. It activates the sympathetic nervous system's well-known fight-or-flight response, which includes surges of adrenaline and cortisol (the hormones that send glycogen to the muscles for an instant energy boost) that speed up heart and breathing rates and raise blood pressure.

But this response is designed by nature to be a short-term emergency fix. It should fully subside once the danger is passed. But too often stress becomes chronic. Under those conditions, your body's rebuilding process can be diminished or slowed down, and in consequence, your muscle building is slowed or even stopped.

Do not let stress affect your health and quality of life. Fortunately, exercise is an excellent counter to stress and can bring your body back to a state of homeostasis where heart rate, breathing, and other functions are normal. If stress and its partner anxiety try to affect your mind and body between workouts, practice meditation, yoga, and deep breathing.

4. **Too Little or Too Much**

Are you under-exercising or over-exercising?

You may not be achieving your muscular development goals because you are under exercising. The 21-day plans have been designed to work your muscles:

- ➢ in the right frequency (reps)
- ➢ at the right speed (cycles)
- ➢ in the right number of sets

➤ with the right amount of rest between sets

➤ with the requisite rest and recovery time between workouts

If you are not trying to at least reasonably keep up with the plans, the muscular growth you are hoping for will be slower to occur or may not occur at all. Nowhere in life is this expression more relevant: "You get out of it what you put into it." We all have days when things are slow or we miss an occasional workout, but you have the opportunity to build a great physique, if you are prepared to work at it.

Come on, you've got this.

Over exercising causes problems of its own. Exercising too often and too intensely can damage your muscles in a way where they cannot be repaired with rest and recovery. And instead of building bulk, strength and definition, your muscles can atrophy or reduce in size and strength. Follow the plan, and if there is anything that is at the top of the list, it's the rest and recovery days between workouts. Give your body the rest it needs to rebuild what has been broken down within your muscle fibers. Stay close to the limits of reps, sets, and the speed of cycles recommended in the 21-day plans and don't be tempted to jump ahead to the advanced levels prematurely.

If you do end up overworking or overextending yourself, avoid injury and ensure your recovery with rest. If you are able, perform your calisthenics at a slower pace with fewer reps, fewer sets, more time between sets, and three days to recover between workouts.

Aches and pains can, generally, be managed with NSAIDs, or nonsteroidal anti-inflammatories, better known as aspirin, ibuprofen, and naproxen. Acetaminophen, or Tylenol, can also be used.

Injuries, including sprains and strains, are best treated, according to trainers and orthopedists, with RICE, which stands for Rest, Ice, Compression, and Elevation.

Our last chapter takes a look at some of the myths, mistakes, and misunderstandings associated with calisthenics and bodybuilding.

Chapter 9:

Myths and Misconceptions

With all that is published in magazines and on social media, plus what is promised in advertising and what you may hear others saying in gyms and fitness centers, you may not be sure what is true and what is a myth or misconception.

Here are 10 of the most common myths about calisthenics and fitness as well as the facts you need to know to refute them:

Myth 1: The more/harder you train, the bigger the muscles you will build.

It's normal to be excited and anxious. You've started your calisthenics bodybuilding program, and it's going well, so why not ratchet up the intensity and frequency of the workouts for faster, better results? You know the answer from the previous chapters, but just to repeat it: Overuse of your muscles and not allowing enough time for recovery between workouts will not allow your muscles to grow and may even lead to atrophy or muscle tissue loss. Plus, overdoing it can be a recipe for injuries. Stick to the pacing of the 21-day plans and do not punish your muscles with too much work and not enough rest.

Myth 2: You should feel pain every day after each calisthenics workout.

Some day-after-workout pain is normal and is generally not a concern; it may give you a satisfying reminder that you had a good workout the day before. But pain that is intense or discomforting or that lasts for two or three days is a sign that you are working too hard with too many reps or not enough time between sets. As you condition, there should only be muscular pain on occasional days; pain that is not intense or long lasting. Be alert to joint pains, and be sure you are performing each movement correctly.

Myth 3: Your dietary practice is less important than taking supplements.

We humans evolved over many thousands of years by eating a diversity of natural, unprocessed foods, and there is no precedent for us to ignore a good, balanced diet and try to get our nutrients from highly processed and intensely concentrated supplements. A supplement that promises pumped-up, bulkier muscles in a short time is making false and misleading claims. You may consider whey protein supplements, since getting 100 grams of protein from diet alone can be tough, but your priority should be a quality overall diet. There are also food-based shakes and beverages available at supermarkets, which provide 20 to 30 grams of protein. (See chapter 2 for the full rundown on nutrition.)

Myth 4: Once your workouts slow or stop, your muscle turns to fat.

Muscle is composed of protein, which is a complex molecule, constructed from 20 amino acids, including nine we can only get from foods we eat. As we exercise and damage the muscle fibers, they respond by using protein and amino acids to rebuild. If we begin to slow or even stop our workouts, the muscles will slowly reduce in size. It is physically impossible for muscle to turn to fat, which is chemically composed of free fatty acids. But when exercise slows and caloric intake increases, you can gain weight, which is stored in your body as fat.

Myth 5: You can get rid of belly fat by working your core, especially your abdominals.

While it's true that core exercises will harden and define abdominal muscles, it is not possible to "spot reduce" or burn off fat deposits by exercising. There is only one way to get that fat off your gut and reveal that six-pack hiding behind it: lose weight. And the best way to lose weight steadily is to combine your bodyweight calisthenics workouts with a responsible diet that reduces your caloric intake and the amount of food you eat, especially refined carbohydrates. Also, avoid the empty calories of sugar, watch the fats you eat, and add more protein to your diet to build muscle and keep you feeling fuller longer.

Myth 6: Older people should not exercise too hard or too often.

People of all ages benefit from regular exercise, especially as they grow older. Exercise is good for your muscles, and that includes your heart. Getting your heart to pump harder by gradually warming up and then increasing to a steady, rhythmic pace and sustaining it for 20, 30, or more minutes for several days a week (or more) can keep your heart strong and your arteries open. Practicing calisthenics, as prescribed in our 21-day plans, will build and maintain strength, improve flexibility, and help prevent injuries. Cardio training will optimize heart health, too.

Myth 7: Calisthenics can't really build big muscles.

This all depends on what you consider big muscles. If your goal is to look like an Olympic weightlifter, that means you will have to train like an Olympic weightlifter, working with incredibly heavy weights over several years of, frankly, brutal training. But if your goal is to have the well-developed muscle size, definition, and strength of an athlete, then calisthenics is the ideal exercise routine for you. If you want to see where a good calisthenics program can take you, look instead at Olympic gymnasts.

Myth 8: Calisthenics is only good for certain body types.

There is a misconception that calisthenics mostly benefits those with slender physiques and not people with heavier or broader builds. While it is true that physique types respond and build muscle differently, calisthenics can work effectively for all body types. Lightweight builds seem to achieve the gymnast's physique and good definition faster but don't tend to add much bulk. Heavier builds benefit from their extra body weight providing more resistance, so they bulk up more readily and increase strength faster. Most of us are in-between these extremes and can build both muscle mass and good definition through calisthenics.

Myth 9: The upper body is the area of greatest importance to develop.

We're all impressed when we see big biceps, triceps, shoulders, and, of course, well-developed pectoral muscles of the upper chest. But the core and lower body muscles are of equal or even greater importance, so you need to focus on working the total body. The core muscles include the abdominals, the back, and the lower back muscles. A strong core gives great overall strength and helps prevent injury. You also want to strengthen the hip flexors, the quads, the hamstrings, and the calves, since they hold you up and carry you forward for over 2,000 miles a year on average.

Myth 10: You don't need to do all of the exercises in perfect form to bulk up and get stronger.

It's all up to you: Your results will follow the principle of *getting out of it what you put into it*. So, the better you perform the exercises and complete the routine of the nine calisthenics that are included in the 21-day plans, the more impressive your results will be. The nine exercises were selected to work all of your muscle groups to ensure a complete body workout. Your form and procedure will determine the quality of the calisthenics exercises, so the more fully you perform each exercise, the faster you will see results.

Conclusion

This book was written with the objective of helping anyone at any level achieve the muscular physique and overall physical condition of their dreams. By choosing to read and follow the instructions in this book, you have made a commitment and an investment in yourself, so congratulations for taking this first, important step. Know that:

- ➤ You have committed yourself to finally getting into the shape you have always wanted but just never found the time or had the motivation to accomplish before.
- ➤ You understand that it will take less than an hour for as few as three days a week to achieve your goals.
- ➤ You are ready to take on the challenge.
- ➤ You are making the most important investment of your life, supporting your health, strength, and longevity.
- ➤ You have the right path forward to perform the bodyweight calisthenics that have been carefully chosen for optimal results; just nine exercises in 21-day plans that will take you from basic to

advanced, building solid muscle every step of the way.

➤ You are aware of the importance of two additional factors that will help you achieve your strength and fitness goals: choosing a healthy, balanced, natural, and unprocessed diet and avoiding the wrong foods.

➤ You will practice cardiovascular conditioning to keep your heart and circulatory system in good health while keeping your weight down as you trade unwanted body fat for lean muscle mass.

Never underestimate your potential. Despite any doubts or uncertainties you may have, you are already stronger than you realize. And now, you are on your way to grow stronger with bigger, better-defined muscles and a huge surge in your overall physical ability. You have the undeniable right to grow stronger and look better. You deserve to be healthy and physically fit so that you can build your self-esteem as you become confident in the knowledge that you have the strength to accomplish whatever you set your mind to.

You can look forward to the support and respect of others, who will turn to you for leadership, knowing that you have both the physical strength and stamina of a finely conditioned athlete. You are approaching the day when you can say, whatever the challenge:

"I've got this. I'm in control of the situation. I'll get it done."

Please leave honest feedback about your impressions and thoughts about this book so that we can keep on making improvements to ensure this is the best source of instruction and motivation for all who want to develop bigger muscles and achieve greater strength through bodyweight calisthenics. If this book met or exceeded your expectations, please leave us a top rating so that others will know this is the right book for them.

In wishing you health, success, and personal fulfillment, consider and believe what we know to be unquestionably true:

> **"You are stronger, fitter, and tougher than when you started, and that is certainly something!"**

- Daily Jay

Reference List

Ajani, L. (2020, June 2). How to build muscle at home. *WikiHow.* https://www.wikihow.com/Build-Muscle-at-Home

Antranik. (2017, January 11). How to do horizontal incline rows with minimal equipment. *YouTube.com.* https://www.youtube.com/watch?v=rloXYB8M3vU

Avatar Nutrition (2020). The science behind muscle growth. *Medium.com.* https://medium.com/@avatarnutrition/the-science-behind-muscle-growth-a1b5e9cba225

Bodyweight training and workouts. (2020). School of Calisthenics. Retrieved from https://schoolofcalisthenics.com/

Buff Dude Workouts. (2017, December 7). How to perform chin-ups. *YouTube.com.* https://www.youtube.com/watch?v=brhRXlOhsAM&t=26s

Buff Dudes Workouts. (2017, July 18). How to perform diamond push-ups. *YouTube.com.*

https://www.youtube.com/watch?v=ZR5U3sb-KeE

Build insane muscle mass using only your bodyweight. (2020). Bodyweight Training Arena Retrieved from https://bodyweighttrainingarena.com/workout-how-to-build-insane-muscle-mass-just-with-bodyweight/

Calisthenic Movement (2016, June 16). The perfect push-up - do it right! YouTube.com. https://www.youtube.com/watch?v=IODxDxX7oi4&t=48s

Calisthenic Movement (2016, September 8). The perfect pull-up - do it right! YouTube.com. https://www.youtube.com/watch?v=eGo4IYlbE5g

Calisthenics Movement. (2017, August 10). Ultimate push-up | can you do it? *YouTube.com.* https://www.youtube.com/watch?v=KIEAbfk4cQU

Calculate your basal metabolic rate (BMR) (2020). Retrieved from https://www.bodybuilding.com/fun/bmr_calculator.htm

Cardio exercise, Good for more than your heart. (2020). WebMD. Retrieved from https://www.webmd.com/fitness-exercise/ss/slideshow-cardio-exercise-good-for-more-than-heart?ecd=wnl_spr_091020&ctr=wnl-spr-091020_nsl-Bodymodule_Position6&mb=MukfT6opS3AxbF5kSEwI0ng0WleHxvIqssh%40W36l9r4%3d

Chertoff, J. (2019, November 12). How to add compound exercises to your workout routine. *Healthline.* https://www.healthline.com/health/fitness-exercise/compound-exercises

Creveling, M. (2020, April 15). The best bodyweight exercises you can do at home. *Health.* https://www.health.com/fitness/bodyweight-exercises

Davies, D. (2020, July 28). Build serious muscle with these at-home bodyweight exercises and workouts. *Men's Health.* https://www.menshealth.com/uk/building-muscle/a756325/10-best-bodyweight-exercises-for-men/

Eastman, H. (2018, February 28). The ultimate beginner's guide to calisthenics. *Bodybuilding.com.* https://www.bodybuilding.com/content/the-ultimate-beginners-guide-to-calisthenics.html

FitnessFAQs. (2017, November 23). Straight vs. parallel bar dips | which is better? *YouTube.com.*

https://www.youtube.com/watch?v=2IUoEAzjZqY

FitnessFAQs: (2017, October 12). The worst ab training mistakes. *YouTube.com.* https://www.youtube.com/watch?v=QyVq5oUBpss

Gunnars, K. (2019, June 13). 50 foods that are super healthy. *Healthline.* https://www.healthline.com/nutrition/50-super-healthy-foods

Gunnars, K. (2018, May 7). 5 simple rules for amazing health. *Healthline.* https://www.healthline.com/nutrition/5-simple-rules-for-amazing-health?slot_pos=article_1&utm_source=Sailthru%20Email&utm_medium=Email&utm_campaign=generalhealth&utm_content=2020-09-10&apid=25264436

Herring, R. (2019, April 8). Recuperation and muscular growth! *Bodybuilding.com.* https://www.bodybuilding.com/content/recuperation-and-muscular-growth.html

Holland, T. (2016, August 31). How-to | squats for beginners. *Bowflex/YouTube.com.* https://www.youtube.com/watch?v=aclHkVaku9U

Hybrid Athlete. (2012, August 31). Lateral lunge. *YouTube.com*.
https://www.youtube.com/watch?v=gwWv7aPcD88

Jackson, D. (2020). Building muscle with calisthenics. *School of Calisthenics*.
https://schoolofcalisthenics.com/2019/08/12/building-muscle-with-calisthenics/

Kamb, S. (2020, March 17). The 42 best bodyweight exercises. *Nerd Fitness*.
https://www.nerdfitness.com/blog/the-42-best-bodyweight-exercises-the-ultimate-guide-for-working-out-anywhere/

Kavadlo, D. (2017, June 6). How to build a calisthenics body. *BodyBuilding*.
https://www.bodybuilding.com/content/how-to-build-a-calisthenics-body.html

Keet, L. (2020, September 5). Calisthenics training mistakes with Lee Downing Keet. *Red Delta Project*.
https://reddeltaproject.com/calisthenics-training-mistakes-w-lee-downing-keet/

Kerksick, C., Wilborn, C., et al. (2018, August 1) ISSN exercise and sports nutrition review update: research and recommendations. *Journal of the International Society of Sports Nutrition*.
https://jissn.biomedcentral.com/articles/10.1186/s12970-018-0242-y

Kravitz, L., Kwon, Y.S. (2004). How do muscles grow? *University of New Mexico.* https://www.unm.edu/~lkravitz/Article%20folder/musclesgrowLK.html

Leech, J. (2018, September 14). 11 proven benefits of olive oil. *Healthline.* https://www.healthline.com/nutrition/11-proven-benefits-of-olive-oil

Legumes and pulses. (2020). Harvard T.H. Chan School of Public Health. Retrieved from https://www.hsph.harvard.edu/nutritionsource/legumes-pulses/

Leonard, J. (2018, September 18). What are the benefits of protein powder? *Medical News Today.* https://www.medicalnewstoday.com/articles/323093

Lewis, A. (2020, September 27). 3 muscle mass building myths destroyed. *New Motivation Coaching.* https://newmotivationcoaching.com/workouts/3-muscle-mass-building-myths-destroyed/

Lieberman, B., Tucker, A. (2017, October 3). 53 bodyweight exercises you can do at home. *Self.* https://www.self.com/gallery/bodyweight-exercises-you-can-do-at-home

Lumsden, B. (2019, August 26). Importance of sleep for muscle growth. *Relentless Gains.*

https://relentlessgains.com/importance-of-sleep-for-muscle-growth/

Merrick, T. (2018, May 6). Bodyweight row tutorial. *YouTube.com.* https://www.youtube.com/watch?v=PGcTxvw6-lo

Michael, Yannick. (2020, August 3). Calisthenics pull workout routine. *Calisthenics Family.* https://calisthenics-family.com/articles/calisthenics-pull-workout-routine/

Nunez, K. (2019, June 24). The best core exercises for all fitness levels. *Healthline.* https://www.healthline.com/health/best-core-exercises

Peale, N.V. (1955). The power of positive thinking. *Good Reads.* https://www.goodreads.com/work/quotes/1121350-the-power-of-positive-thinking

Petra, A. (2019, April 8). 13 habits linked to a long life (backed by science. *Healthline.* https://www.healthline.com/nutrition/13-habits-linked-to-a-long-life

Pigmie. (2017, September 24). Tucked planche positions fix. *YouTube.com.* https://www.youtube.com/watch?v=iT1q1Ff02mk

Quinn, E. (2020, August 29). Scientific rules that lead to physical fitness. *Very Well Fit.* https://www.verywellfit.com/the-6-scientific-rules-you-must-follow-to-get-fit-3120111

Quinn, E. (2020, March 25). Signs and symptoms of overtraining syndrome in athletes. *Very Well Fit.* https://www.verywellfit.com/overtraining-syndrome-and-athletes-3119386

Quinn, E. (2020, February 13). Importance of rest and recovery after your exercise. *Very Well Fit.* https://www.verywellfit.com/the-benefits-of-rest-and-recovery-after-exercise-3120575

Reed, K. (June 18, 2018). How do muscles grow: the science of muscle growth explained. *Positive Health Wellness.* https://www.positivehealthwellness.com/fitness/how-do-muscles-grow-the-science-of-muscle-growth-explained/

Rizzo, J. (2012, June 12), How to do a leg raise | Ab workout. *Howcast/YouTube.com.* https://www.youtube.com/watch?v=l4kQd9eWclE

Rizzo, J. (2012, June 11), How to do a side plank | Ab workout. *Howcast/YouTube.com.* https://www.youtube.com/watch?v=NXr4Fw8q60o

Robson, D. (2020, July 8). The importance of sleep. *Bodybuilder.com*. https://www.bodybuilding.com/content/the-importance-of-sleep.html

Rogers, P. (2020, August 3). The best lower body strength exercises. *Very Well Fit*. *https://www.verywellfit.com/best-lowerbody-weight-training-exercises-3498517*

Salyer, J. (2016, December 19). 5 Examples of isometric exercises for static strength training. *Healthline*. https://www.healthline.com/health/fitness-exercise/isometric-exercises

Singh, E. (2019, May 20). Beginner advice from 5 calisthenics experts. *Warrior Academy*. https://warrioracademyhk.com/beginner-advice-from-5-calisthenics-experts-includes-al-kavadlo/

Teagarden, C. (2020, July 12). How to do dips at home (without a dip bar). *YouTube.com*. https://www.youtube.com/watch?v=isikOOF0W3k

Tober, J. (2016, November 12) Calf raises - the easiest way to instantly get better athletically. *YouTube.com*. https://www.youtube.com/watch?v=TZrBb5M1CdM

TPindell Fitness. (2015, September 28). How to do Superman exercises. *YouTube.com*. https://www.youtube.com/watch?v=VUT1RHyMEuc

The 30 best bodyweight exercises for men. (n.d). Men's Journal. Retrieved from https://www.mensjournal.com/health-fitness/the-30-best-bodyweight-exercises-for-men/

Ultimate list of compound exercises - 104+ exercises. (2020). Bodyweight Tribe. Retrieved from https://bodyweighttribe.com/list-of-compound-exercises/

Weiner, Z. (2020, June 2). Trainers say the Superman exercise is the best way to work your obliques. *Well and Good*. https://www.wellandgood.com/superman-exercises/

What is a serving? (2020). Retrieved from *Heart.org*. https://www.heart.org/en/health-topics/caregiver-support/what-is-a-serving

Wilson, K.L. (2018, December 12). How much carbs, fat and protein should you eat daily to lose weight? *SFGate*. https://healthyeating.sfgate.com/much-carbs-fat-protein-should-eat-daily-lose-weight-6278.html

Yetman, D. (2020, May 28). What muscle groups are best to workout together? *Healthline*. https://www.healthline.com/health/exercise-fitness/muscle-groups-to-workout-together

Image Sources

Fig. 1 (2020). Retrieved from https://pixabay.com/images/search/push%20up/

Fig. 2 (2016). Retrieved from https://www.youtube.com/watch?v=eGo4IYlbE5g. Screenshot by author.

Fig. 3 (2017). Retrieved from https://www.youtube.com/watch?v=brhRXlOhsAM/. Screenshot by author.

Fig. 4 (2016). Retrieved from https://www.youtube.com/watch?v=IODxDxX7oi4&feature=youtu.be. Screenshot by author.

Fig. 5 (2020). Retrieved from https://www.youtube.com/watch?v=isikOOF0W3k. Screenshot by author.

Fig. 6 (2012). Retrieved from https://www.youtube.com/watch?v=l4kQd9eWclE. Screenshot by author.

Fig. 7 (2012). https://www.youtube.com/watch?v=NXr4Fw8q60o. Screenshot by author.

Fig. 8 (2015). Retrieved from https://www.youtube.com/watch?v=VUT1RHyMEuc. Screenshot by author.

Fig. 9 (2016). Retrieved from https://www.youtube.com/watch?v=aclHkVaku9U. Screenshot by author.

Fig. 10 (2016). Retrieved from https://www.youtube.com/watch?v=TZrBb5M1CdM. Screenshot by author.

Fig. 11 (2017). Retrieved from https://www.youtube.com/watch?v=QyVq5oUBpss. Screenshot by author.

Fig. 12 (2017). Retrieved from https://www.youtube.com/watch?v=rloXYB8M3vU. Screenshot by author.

Fig. 13 (2018). Retrieved from https://www.youtube.com/watch?v=PGcTxvw6-lo. Screenshot by author.

Fig. 14 (2017). Retrieved from https://www.youtube.com/watch?v=ZR5U3sb-KeE. Screenshot by author.

Fig. 15 (2016). Retrieved from https://www.youtube.com/watch?v=h0HjqYRlXYg. Screenshot by author.

Fig. 16 (2017). Retrieved from https://www.youtube.com/watch?v=KIEAbfk4cQU. Screenshot by author.

Fig. 17 (2017). Retrieved from https://www.youtube.com/watch?v=2IUoEAzjZqY. Screenshot by author.

Fig. 18 (2017). Retrieved from https://www.youtube.com/watch?v=2IUoEAzjZqY. Screenshot by author.

Fig. 19 (2017). Retrieved from https://www.youtube.com/watch?v=iT1q1Ff02mk. Screenshot by author.

Fig. 20 (2012). Retrieved from https://www.youtube.com/watch?v=gwWv7aPcD88. Screenshot by author.

www.ingramcontent.com/pod-product-compliance
Lightning Source LLC
Chambersburg PA
CBHW020906080526
44589CB00011B/462